CW00485431

Psoriatic Arthr

Psoriatic Arthritis treatme strategies.

Psoriatic Arthritis causes, outlook, diet, therapies, supplements and home remedies.

by

Colin Cumberstone

Table of Contents

Chapter 1: Introduction

Seeking the right treatment for Psoriatic Arthritis (PA) can be a very hectic quest and even after a lifelong search the perfect cure is still an illusion. There are a lot of things that can be done at home to help you with PA. There are several factors in the environment and modulating them slightly can bring significant relief to your PA. Some of these don't even require any help, as you can do it yourself. Let me explain it with one example here.

PA flare-ups are very common during changes in weather conditions and temperatures around you. Try to evaluate the best temperature for you during weather changes. Stay home around that ideal temperature and avoid flare-ups. Abrupt temperature changes can be avoided by a gradual exposure to warmer or colder weather variation. Set your ideal temperature both in the office and at home. Spend less time outdoors during the weather change. This is just one example to give you an idea about the book and there are many more practical tips in this book to provide you effective and swift relief from the pain and agony of PA. Self-assessment can be initiated by asking yourself the following simple questions.

-How self-conscious do you feel about your PA?

-How helpless do you feel regarding your PA?

-How angry or frustrated do you feel regarding your PA?

-To what extent does your PA interfere with your capacity to enjoy life?

-How much physical pain or soreness do you feel?

A clear self-assessment will lead to better implementation of the treatment regimens and tips offered in the following chapters. Most of the tips in this book require a basic understanding of PA and hence we'll start with that.

It is now recognised that psoriatic arthritis is far more common than the previously considered number of 10% of patients with psoriasis. Now it is estimated that more than 30% of all psoriasis patients develop PA. It is debilitating, disabling and progressive in nature. Five different clinical patterns of psoriatic arthritis have been recognised that can coexist with overlapping clinical features. These are:

-1. **Asymmetrical polyarthritis or oligoarthritis**: Found in almost 50% of patients of PA, it is characterised by morning stiffness, distal (DIP) and proximal interphalangeal (PIP) involvement, nail disease and 4 or fewer joints are involved.

-2. **Symmetrical polyarthritis**: It involves the simultaneous development of psoriasis and arthritis.

-3. **Ankylosing spondylitis**: It is easily distinguishable due to progressive lower back pain, morning stiffness, sacroiliac, and axial joint involvement.

-4. **DIP joint disease**: It is characterised by nail and joint involvement (DIP) predominates.

-5. **Arthritis mutilans**: It is the most destructive form of arthritis, telescoping, joint lysis, typically in phalanges, and metacarpals. Fortunately, it is also very rare.

The first three types of PA account for almost 95% cases of PA, the last two are rare with less than 5% incidence. Understanding these different scenarios can help in the prevention of disability and progression of PA. This is particularly important with the latest medications currently available, which have been shown to prevent further joint damage.

Like any other chronic arthritic disease, psoriatic arthritis also varies in the severity of its symptoms. Knowledge of the factors responsible for this variation can help you to manage it better. They can be divided into two groups.

-1. Factors worsening PA

-2. Factors prolonging the duration of therapy-induced remission

The information about the first group is much more common and patients can find it on their own via personal experience. The information about the second group is comprised of favourable conditions and treatments that facilitate disease remission and control. It is this second group that this book explains in detail, just like the example shared in previous paragraphs. Following is a brief list of factors that can worsen the psoriatic arthritis:

* Emotional stress

* Activation of local cellular immunity:

- Immune activity in affected joints,

- Joint infections,

* Systemic immunological activation or alteration:

- Hypersensitivity to any treatment component,

- HIV infection,

* Systemic drugs (through pharmacological actions):

- Corticosteroids,

- Interferons,

- Lithium,

- Antimalarials (chloroquine, hydroxychloroquine, quinacrine, quinidine),

- Beta-Blockers (adrenergic receptor antagonists: many different agents both selective and non-selective) Non-steroidal anti-inflammatory drugs (NSAID's),

- Angiotensin-converting enzyme (ACE) inhibitors,

- Gemfibrozil and a number of other drugs in case reports.

A physician must consider all the above aspects when assessing patient condition and formulating the best treatment regimen for the patient. Being a patient, you can make his/her job easy if you know and understand several key factors prior to seeing your physician. For a head start, you can focus on some basic aspects during a doctor-patient session. You can expect discussion on symptoms, diagnosis, hereditary aspects, systemic manifestations of arthritis, exacerbating and favourable factors, response to past treatments, range of therapeutic options, chronic long-term disease effects, psychological ramifications and optimism for tomorrow as new therapies are in the pipeline.

Talking of optimism, I must reiterate that this book has plenty to offer when it comes to the "DO IT YOURSELF" part of the treatment that can go a long way in normalising your life while minimising the debilitating effects of psoriatic arthritis. Here is a brief mention of some of the natural treatment options you'll come across in this book in detail.

- Complementary Therapies:

Specific Treatments

- Ice T,

- Fish Oil Supplements,

- Avo-Kale Arthritis Arrester,

- RICE: Rest, Ice, Compression, Elevation,

- Turmeric-Ginger Inflammation Fighter,

- Muscle-Boosting Beet and Tart Cherry Tonic,

- Açai Smoothie,

- Anti-Inflammatory Pineapple-Ginger Salsa,

- Herbal Pain-Relieving Poultice.

Lifestyle Tips & Modifications:

- Consider Magnets,

- Stretch three times a week,

- Castor oil pack,

- Listen to your body,

- Traveling Tips,

- Mild Yoga,

- Aloe Vera,

- Chinese Herbs,

- Spa Treatments,

- Balneo-therapy,

- Tai chi,

- Exercise.

Together we'll explore some very exciting natural treatment options for managing psoriatic arthritis successfully. Enjoy the book.

Chapter 2: What is Psoriatic Arthritis?

Psoriatic arthritis is a long-lasting disease considered as a form of inflammation of the skin (psoriasis) and joints (inflammatory arthritis). Arthritis is particularly the inflammation of joints. The main symptom is joint-pain, which increases with age and other related factors. Similarly, *Psoriatic arthritis* is a type of arthritic inflammation that particularly means joint inflammation. The inflammation of arthritis sources swelling, pain, arduousness, and redness in the joints. It usually arises in 15 per cent of patients who have the skin disease called psoriasis. The start of psoriatic arthritis generally happens in the fourth and fifth decades of life. Males and females are affected equally. This type of arthritis can affect any joint in the body but symptoms vary from patient to patient. Treatments available for this disease are usually successful for most people. This type of arthritis can affect any joint in the body; it can also affect multiple joints. For example, it may affect one or both knees. It can affect toes and fingers and they become swollen. Fingers and toenails can also be affected badly. Psoriatic arthritis is a chronic arthritis. In some patients it is as simple as usual cuts. In other patients, it is a permanent disease and can cause joint damage if not treated properly. For most of the patients, appropriate treatment leads to proper pain relief and joint mobility.

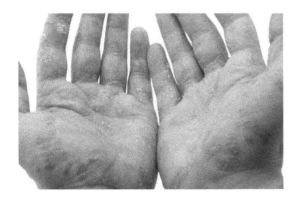

Definitions for Psoriatic Arthritis

(1) - "Psoriatic arthritis is a severe form of arthritis accompanied by inflammation, psoriasis of the skin or nails, and a negative test for rheumatoid factor—called also psoriasis arthropathica." – Merriam & Webster medical dictionary.

(2) – "It is a form of arthritis that affects some percentage of people who have psoriasis — a condition that features red patches of skin topped with silvery scales." – Online medical dictionary.

Psoriatic Arthritis-Fast Facts:

- Psoriatic arthritis is a chronic disease in the form of inflammation of the skin,

- Almost 10 to 15% of people with psoriasis also develop inflammation of joints (psoriatic arthritis),

- The first appearance of the skin disease can be separated from the joint inflammation,

- Psoriatic arthritis can also cause inflammation of the spine (spondyloarthropathies),

- To avoid joint damage early diagnose is important,

- Family history does matter because people having patients in the family have higher chances of suffering from this disease.

The relationship between Psoriasis & Psoriatic Arthritis

Arthritis causes inflammation, joint swelling and pain, and may lead to permanent defect and damage if not treated. Whereas in psoriatic arthritis, additionally, patches or plaques of scaly and inflamed skin occur. Almost 30 per cent of people suffering from psoriasis develop psoriatic arthritis. Usually skin symptoms of psoriasis appear before psoriatic arthritis develops. It is possible, however, for psoriatic arthritis symptoms to take months and years to appear before any skin cuts grow.

Both psoriasis and psoriatic arthritis are mainly caused by an exaggerated immune system response. In the case of your skin, this causes cells to grow too quickly.

There does not seem to be a link between where the peeling skin patches from psoriasis are located and which joints are affected by psoriatic arthritis. For example, you could have skin cuts and damage on both your fingers, but your finger joints could be unaffected by psoriatic arthritis. In the same way, psoriatic arthritis could cause swelling of the toes without any redness on the feet.

In fact, some patients have arthritis more than 20 years before psoriasis eventually appears. On the other hand, patients can have psoriasis for over 20 years prior to the development of arthritis or prior to the ultimate diagnosis of psoriatic arthritis.

Psoriatic Arthritis & Other Spondyloarthritides

Spondyloarthritides particularly refers to the disease that causes the inflammation of spine. In other words, this type of arthritis affects the spine.

There are some other types of arthritis that fall under the spondyloarthritides. These include:

- *Ankylosing spondylitis*: causes inflammation of joints in the spine.

- *Psoriatic arthritis*: related to the skin condition psoriasis.
- Reactive arthritis: occurs as a result of infection in the body.
- Enteropathic arthritis: related to inflammatory bowel diseases, such as ulcerative colitis disease. Almost 1 in 10 people develop this type of bowl arthritis.
- Undifferentiated spondyloarthritis: a form of spondyloarthritides that is different from any of the above types.

What treatments are there for Spondyloarthritis?

Your rheumatologist will modify your treatment according to your symptoms and how severe your condition is. There is no best way of predicting exact treatment for one's disease. Your doctor may need to test several different treatments before finding the one that suits you best and may include:

* Physiotherapy exercises, to keep the joints flexible and improve posture
* Medicines, such as: painkillers, e.g. paracetamol.
* Non-steroidal anti-inflammatory drugs (NSAIDs)
* Corticosteroid medicines or injections
* Disease-modifying anti-rheumatic drugs (DMARDs)
* Biological DMARDs, such as tumour necrosis factor (TNF) medicines.

Chapter 3: What Causes Psoriatic Arthritis?

The human body is prone to numerous health complications and diseases. Whenever we are ill, one or more organs are set to perform incorrectly. Medical science knows several diseases that affect only one organ and have simple treatment options available. On the other hand, several illnesses involve multiple disorders and require a complex approach. We have many examples of such cases. For example, most of the liver and heart related disorders can affect more than one organ in the body. Diabetes and hypertension are prime examples. Arthritis and some of its subtypes like Psoriatic arthritis can target more than one area. Psoriatic arthritis is known to involve the two most critical organs; bones (particularly joints) and skin. Multiple causes can lead to both arthritis and its subtype Psoriatic arthritis.

Causes of Psoriatic Arthritis

There are multiple findings on the causes of PA:

- It is believed that factors like genetic makeup, environment and immune system play an important role. It is found that 50% of these patients have a gene marker HLA-B27 found.

- It is also believed that main risk factors causing psoriatic arthritis are family history, age between 30 – 50 years and men are more likely to be a victim of this disease than women. Researchers found that 40% of patients have close relatives like siblings or parents with psoriasis or psoriatic arthritis.

- It is also believed that people with some trauma or stress will develop psoriatic arthritis if these people have psoriasis.

Clinical Features of Psoriatic Arthritis

Generally, there are five major clinical features of psoriatic arthritis:

(1) – Symmetrical polyarthritis (30-50% of cases) is the most common presentation of psoriatic arthritis,

(2) – Asymmetrical oligoarthritis is also a presentation,

(3) – Distal interphalangeal (DIP) joint involvement is associated with nail psoriasis,

(4) – Arthritis mutilans is known by resorption of the phalanges, and

(5) – Axial arthritis might differ characteristically from ankylosing spondylitis, the prototypical HLA-B27-associated spondyloarthritis.

There is radiographic evidence of sacroiliitis with lower back pain and inflammation that it is normally asymmetrical, or can be asymptomatic or spondylitis which may occur without sacroiliitis and may affect any level of the spine in a non-contiguous manner.

There are few non-popular conditions as well. These conditions are listed below:

(1) – Nail involvement classified as onycholysis,

(2) – Nail pitting,

(3) – Dactylitis,

(4) – Diffuse swelling of the entire digit likely due to a combination of both arthritis and tenosynovitis,

(5) – Extra-articular manifestations.

Radiographic Features of Psoriatic Arthritis

The most common radiological feature of erosive change with bone proliferation is a predominantly distal distribution. The disease commonly involves the hands and feet. It can also affect sacroiliac joints and the spine. Knees, elbows, ankles, and shoulders are also involved but to a lesser extent.

In hands and feet, the pattern of distribution may be that of symmetric or asymmetric. Imaging findings include:

- Pencil in cup deformations, enthesitis and marginal bone erosions,

14

- Joint subluxation or inter-phalangeal ankylosis,

- Bone proliferation results in an irregular, "fuzzy" appearance to the bone around the affected joint,

- Periostitis - may appear as a periosteal layer of new bone, or as irregular thickening of the cortex itself,

- Dactylitis - which can present as a "sausage digit" which refers to soft tissue swelling of a whole digit; ultrasound examination of a sausage digit demonstrates underlying synovitis and tenosynovitis.

Chapter 4: Other effects of Psoriatic Arthritis

Psoriatic arthritis is a lifelong disease, hence it is necessary to maintain good joint health so as keep the joints flexible and increase their mobility. Psoriatic arthritis not only affects individuals in terms of physical health but it also leads to emotional and psychosocial impairment. Furthermore, the quality of life is affected and such individuals are overburdened with lifelong financial crisis.

Functional & Emotional Impact

Psoriatic arthritis being a chronic, lifelong disease has an emotional toll on an individual's life. They need support, both psychological and emotional, from their family and friends. The burden of the disease makes it difficult for such individuals to seek emotional support. The pain, stiffness and fatigue associated with psoriatic arthritis causes them to shy away from asking anyone for help or for that matter to be positive and be active in their daily routine. The psychosocial distress causes people with psoriatic arthritis to have reduced life goals and satisfaction. Due to the psychosocial distress the quality of life is affected, mentally, emotionally and physically. There is an increase in the other conditions that further make the health of people with psoriatic arthritis worse over time. For example, such individuals may end up having hypertension, heart disease, respiratory system disease or involvement of their gastrointestinal tract. Their bone health is also compromised, which causes the pain to be unbearable.

According to researches and studies, fatigue is the most commonly reported problem that people with psoriatic arthritis suffer from. It has been redeemed as the major factor that causes disability and deteriorates the physical and mental status.

Some individuals even suffer from negative thinking leading to anxiety and irritability. It is important for such people to express their emotions. Whenever the disease flare-ups occur, the patient may feel depressed and upset, making them unable to handle themselves or carry out their daily functions. The feelings of anxiety lead to lack of sleep, causing fatigue and stress on the body. The fear of the disease is enough to cause them to stay isolated from their family and friends. Sometimes it is possible that others may not be able to help them, as they may feel frightened by the disease. In addition to this, the patients are forced out of their relationships as people around them start to avoid them. Thus, the emotional stress along with pain and discomfort makes the illness difficult to be handled on their own. This disease has a massive impact on a person, resulting in disability and lower quality of life. Such stressors increase the burden of the disease and further make the condition worse. It may result in lack of sleep, inability to exercise, increased irritability, withdrawal from daily life, appetite changes and depression. Poor mental health may lead to depression and/or anxiety. Depression may be classified when patients with psoriatic arthritis may feel withdrawn, fatigued and avoid socialising. They might stay at home all the time, have trouble concentrating or even have difficulty in getting out of bed. There may be subtle signs of suicide or feelings of worthlessness. It is advised for people experiencing such emotions to talk to their doctors, so that their treatment can be reviewed.

Knowing that there is no immediate way or therapy for people with psoriatic arthritis to feel better, it is considered important for them to take appropriate measures to deal with their disease. If these emotions are not dealt with, they may result in having negative thoughts to losing their personal goals and relationships. They must understand that letting go and not exercising or for that matter not taking their medications on time can lead to an increase in the progression of their disease. All in all the exercise may not only help ease their pain and joint stiffness, it also has been known to increase and regulate the hormonal balance, boosting their moods especially if they are feeling down or having low moods.

Apart from the family support, social support is also important. Studies have proven that a strong group be it of family, friends or a support group helps in coping with psoriatic arthritis. In some cases, it has been found to improve compliance with medications as well as exercise, if they have failed on their own. The motivation to deal with the flare-ups is the key factor to dealing with psoriatic arthritis. Expressing the guilt, fear, ignorance and insecurity and receiving comfort from the surrounding people has demonstrated to have good results. If they have a place where they can feel safe to let go of their negativities and be able to talk and discuss whatever is on their mind about the disease; that way a person may start to feel emotionally secure and stable enough to deal with their disease.

There is an increased sense of control, better compliance with medications and exercise with increased life span as a result of a strong and motivating social support group. The positive feedback from the people around can lessen the burden of negativity as well as improving the coping skills. So, when there is a moment of crisis, a person may not feel alone and talk to someone who can help them overcome their painful crises.

Seeking medical or group therapies and talking to your doctor about coping with psoriatic arthritis are considered beneficial in the long-term. The early help ensures that a person feels better being able to handle him/herself. This brings steady performance both in daily routine as well as work routine.

Chapter 5: Non-drug Therapy

Regarding Psoriatic arthritis, multiple triggers are considered responsible for flaring up the disease, and making it worse with the passage of time. Amongst other therapies, non-drug therapy including lifestyle modifications and other home treatments can help manage psoriatic arthritis. The lifestyle changes are necessary so that the progression of the disease can be halted and pain can be managed in order to carry out daily activities. You may talk to your doctor regarding the various therapies, which may include hot or cold treatments. Using a simple heating pad or a simple ice pack can reduce the intensity of your pain and the severity of the swelling of your joints.

In the same manner, using heating pads can help you relax your tense muscles, alleviating pain and the associated stiffness. Such remedies can be used on a day-to-day basis for approximately 30 minutes or so.

Lifestyle changes as per your routine need to be adjusted to help you or someone you know to reduce the wear and tear of joints. Avoid lifting heavy objects, walking at a slow pace, not bending your joints or taking precautions when carrying out your activities can help you cope with the pain better. Therefore, following precautions is equally important in managing psoriatic arthritis. Even resting while doing your daily tasks can help you preserve your stamina and help you relax your joints.

Dietary changes, herbs and supplementation such as fish oil and vitamin D in particular are proven to be beneficial in maintaining a proper balance of your body. Eliminating dairy products, gluten, corn, soy and sugar and whole unprocessed foods have shown to improve the symptoms related to psoriatic arthritis. Overweight individuals may find it hard to tackle their joint problems. The weight of an individual may determine the stress-related joint injury. This is the main reason why you should talk to your doctor about weight reduction as well as a proper dietary plan. A low fat diet, enriched in vegetables and fruits is necessary to maintain a healthy balance. Alcohol, sugar and trans-fats should be avoided, as they are responsible for increasing the inflammatory process in psoriatic arthritis. Physical exercise is as important as the rest of the factors to prevent the joint pain caused by psoriatic arthritis.

Improper use of the joints and lack of exercise can lead to the worsening of the disease, thereby causing muscle weakness. Proper exercise is vital to improve health and flexible joints. A daily exercise routine may help to relieve pain and stiffness of the joints. It is important to select an exercise program that focuses on the range of motions including other strengthening exercises. Low impact aerobics may be considered helpful without stressing the joints and muscles. In the same manner, using a walking aid or shoe inserts help the joints and avoid further stress on the feet, ankles or knees affected by psoriatic arthritis. Similarly, positive changes in your posture at work, home or during leisure time is thought to help relax the joints. Good posture, either sitting or standing and not arching the back is helpful in preserving the joints.

Other treatments like yoga, tai chi, qigong, acupuncture, aromatherapy, physical therapy, swimming and walking in water have been proven useful in patients with psoriatic arthritis. Some people have shown better results in managing their pain under water due to the fact that the buoyancy of the water helps in supporting the joints, releasing the tension of the muscles, strengthening the joints, without stressing their joints, hence protecting them from further damage and maintaining their cardiovascular endurance. Mind endurance exercises have a potent effect on the relaxation of muscles, joints and body. Mind and body therapies are recommended as they help to have a better control of the heart functions, blood pressure and muscle/joint flexibility.

Splinting is another remedy used to support the joints and muscles. It helps to reduce the inflammation of joints and stabilises the joints. However, splinting reduces pain but it has to be removed from time to time so as to restore and improve the mobility of the joints.

Chapter 6: Drug Therapy

Life has a lot to offer. Sometimes life offers joy and other times serious setbacks. Wear and tear, accidental injuries, occasional hard knock, daily hassles, life-threatening microorganisms and worries are all part of life. Fortunately, we possess abundant resources to show resilience against all kinds of setbacks and get back to normal life. Nowadays, doctors are using the latest technology and techniques to treat everyday aliments. We have the access to natural and self-made remedies to fight and prevent illnesses. However, there is also another side to the healing process. You devote yourself completely to the treatment. A patient has to understand that a doctor is not always responsible for the entire treatment process. The patient also has a significant part to play. Additionally, some ailments require combined efforts from both the patient and the doctor. This lesson is more applicable to Psoriatic arthritis patients, where the lifestyle of a patient plays an important part in successfully coping and treatment.

There are a lot of things that a Psoriatic arthritis patient can do. You can opt for home remedies, natural coping options and complimentary treatments. More importantly, motivation and self-assessment are equally important as medications and other medical treatments can be.

A Patient's Story:

I am a Psoriatic arthritis patient and coping with my ailment successfully. Let me begin my story by saying that everyone has a childhood story and so do I. When I was a child, I used to be afraid of a tree. It was on the way to my school. It was dark and gigantic, full of intense and profound fear. Undoubtedly, I was not the only one who feared that tree; a lot of my schoolmates felt the same. I was so afraid of that tree that I used to pray that someone would cut it down. My parents tried to explain to me several times that trees are good for humans but all in vain. Every day, a cloud of thoughts used to strike my mind, and I finally came up with an idea that gave me hope. After that day, I started to paint that tree with colours. Soon it was full of colours and no longer a dark and fearful tree. In fact, it was totally the opposite. I turned my enemy into my friend. After that incident, I learnt that fear can never be a solution. Whenever I face any problem or illness I consider it as that tree from my childhood. Today, I am fighting my illness, coping with symptoms, seeking treatment and living a normal life.

Starting Medication

Psoriatic arthritis is a joint modifying disease that usually occurs during 30-50 years. The choice of medication, course and duration of treatment vary from individual to individual. Your doctor may be the better judge as to which drugs would be helpful in controlling your symptoms of psoriatic arthritis.

One thing that is essential to understand is that psoriatic arthritis can be effectively controlled by the use of appropriate medications, thereby helping to better manage difficult symptoms. But according to the Arthritis Foundation, psoriatic arthritis cannot be cured. If the inflammatory process is controlled or even reduced, the joint pain and swelling will settle, helping a person to lead a near to normal life. Hence preventing further damage and stopping the disease from progression. In addition, lifestyle modifications can help treat the pain, swelling and joint damage.

NSAIDs

Non-steroidal anti-inflammatory drugs are used to control the mild to moderate effects of psoriatic arthritis. Non-steroidal anti-inflammatory drugs such as aspirin, indomethacin, ibuprofen, diclofenac, piroxicam and others have been used to decrease the pain associated with psoriatic arthritis. The mechanism by which these non-steroidal anti-inflammatory drugs act is based upon their action on the inflammatory modulators. The process of inflammation is regulated by the cells that cause damage to the cells and surrounding tissues. These drugs help to decrease the inflammation and joint pain, thus significantly reducing joint stiffness. As the stiffness is reduced, there is a huge improvement in the motion of the joints. Not only the movement gets better but the swelling and redness of the joints as a result of joint inflammation is also vastly improved.

NSAIDs can be obtained over-the-counter but as a safe bet it is better to consult your doctor before starting this therapy. There are some known contraindications and side effects related to the long-term use of non-steroidal anti-inflammatory drugs (NSAIDs), which are considered to injure other vital organs of your body.

Few known side effects of NSAIDs are indigestion, stomach ulcer, increased blood pressure, anaemia, bleeding from your gut, shortness of breath and tiredness. Your doctor may prescribe you some drugs to protect the lining of your stomach so as to avoid stomach pains and bleeding. Other serious side effects are heart failure, heart attack, hypertension, stroke and worsening of inflammatory bowel disease. Then again, not to forget the metabolism of NSAIDs have an adverse effect on the liver and kidneys. Therefore, people suffering from pre-existing heart, liver or kidney disorders have to consult their doctor before planning to start their treatment with these drugs.

Another revolutionary treatment that can be a substitute for NSAIDs is known as cyclooxygenase-2 inhibitors. These COX-2 inhibitors are better than NSAIDs with having fewer effects on the gastrointestinal tract. They have been proven beneficial in treating other forms of arthritis like rheumatoid arthritis and osteoarthritis. Celebrex is one of the many COX-2 inhibitors used for such conditions. They are useful in people who have stomach or acidity problems, as they do not erode the stomach lining. Although, the effect may not be as potent as NSAIDs but their use have been proven to relieve pain and inflammation in psoriatic arthritis patients. COX-2 inhibitors have a disadvantage over

NSAIDs of being expensive in the market. Thus, due to the adverse effects, some of the COX-2 inhibitors were removed from the market while the others were available only on prescription, making them unavailable over the counter.

Steroid therapy

In the year 1952, steroid therapy was initiated to help patients with psoriatic arthritis. Steroids are known for their multiple actions on the body; anti-inflammatory, anti-proliferative, immunosuppressive and vasoconstrictive properties. The mechanism by which steroids act is solely based on binding to the steroid receptor complex. It thereby stimulates gene transcription, further down regulating the inflammatory response. Such inflammatory mediators are then suppressed by steroids inhibiting the immune response that includes vascular dilatation, capillary leaking and skin redness. All in all the total immune activity of the immune cells is decreased so as to stop the damage to the cells, tissues and joints as this exaggerated immune response is the main cause of giving rise to psoriatic lesions on the body, especially in the joints and the skin.

Steroids are not recommended to be used long-term either orally or by injections. The main purpose of steroids is to eliminate the acute or short-term related joint inflammation and swelling. Even if large doses are given, it may lead to the worsening of the psoriatic arthritis. As far evidence postulates, steroidal injections with a low dose near the tendons and around the joints have improved range of motion in such individuals. Topical steroidal application such as ointments, creams, solutions, gels, lotion and sprays are also proven to have a temporary effect in relieving acute pain in psoriatic arthritis.

There are some known side effects that are associated with the continuous use of steroids; they may be as minor as redness, thinning of the skin, increased hair growth and changes in pigmentation to some major ones like bruising, infection of the mouth, acne, rebound flare, eye problems, ulcers, cataracts, growth retardation, pituitary hormonal suppression, electrolyte disturbance, diabetes and other endocrinology related problems. The local effects of steroids are sometimes termed as minor due to the fact that there is minimal absorption of steroids through the application of creams or ointments. After some time, the thinning of the skin due to loss of collagen due to anti-proliferative action of steroids can be reversed. The systemic effects, though not so frequent, can still occur and cause the patients to lose compliance or switch to another option, which might be less toxic compared to steroids. Steroids, when used orally or as injections, have a widespread effect on the human body. It is absorbed in an increased concentration into the bloodstream. Such effects are seen in cases where steroid use has been prolonged, leading to the suppression of the hypothalamic pituitary axis. Other rare syndromes like Cushing syndrome have also been reported. The potency of steroids should always be kept in mind when prescribing them to psoriasis patients.

In children and pregnancy, the use of steroids is still a safety concern. Though it has been found that the use of steroids has improved psoriasis in pregnant patients but the risk of developing abnormalities in the baby is a concerning point for the physicians. In the treatment of pregnant patients with psoriatic arthritis, the benefits should be weighed against the risk of foetal abnormalities that might occur due to the treatment.

Steroids are not used orally to treat psoriatic arthritis instead injections are used for joints that are painful and inflamed.

Steroid injections can be used in supplementation with NSAIDs, physical therapy and supportive devices such as canes and other walking aids. Steroid injections are very useful during flare-ups as it can help to restore muscle and joint movement, thereby decreasing pain and joint stiffness due to inflammation. However, sometimes the long-term use of steroids can lead to the worsening of the disease and an increase in the number of flare-related reactions in people who did not have it before.

Physicians believe that if steroids are to be used, it should be done under strict guidance of the physician.

Other treatments

NSAIDs and steroids by far are the most commonly used medications for preserving joint function in people suffering from psoriatic arthritis. Immunosuppressant drugs, disease modifying drugs, anti-malarial drugs and the recently available anti-tumour necrosis factor agents can be used in people who respond poorly to NSAIDs and steroids. Their side effects are more serious, but these drugs can either be used alone or in combination therapy. Immunosuppressant drugs have been known to cause a massive decline in the production of normal cells of the body, and are considered as the last option for treatment of psoriatic arthritis. Keeping this in mind, the erosions of joints involved in psoriatic arthritis as well as other prognostic factors are necessary to be evaluated upon beginning of such an aggressive treatment.

Newest available drug Otezla (apremilast) is available for having a strong and potent effect on decreasing the inflammation within the cell. It inhibits an enzyme that is responsible for controlling the immune-related response. It may be started as a short-term therapy and continued on achieving its desired effect.

Phototherapy including PUVA, UVB or laser involves ultraviolet light as a treatment for psoriatic arthritis. The only factor that helps is having continuous sessions to achieve the desired effect.

Chapter 7: Current outlook for patients with Psoriatic Arthritis

For the people suffering from psoriatic arthritis, the biggest question is as to the outcome of the disease or the life expectancy and functional capacity. It is evident that psoriatic arthritis is a chronic disease and it does have a huge impact on the quality of life. In most cases, there is pain and impairment mainly during the flare-ups. Therefore, the pain leads to further disability, making it difficult for patients to manage their every day routine. However, it may be mild at times and not causing a lot of problems for the patient. The disease may at times be severe, making it impossible for them to exercise or carry out their daily chores. Lifestyle changes and medications have been proven useful in managing the disease at the same time increasing the life expectancy and lowering the disease progression. There has been no discrimination of the gender or age of people having psoriatic arthritis.

Psoriatic arthritis is not a life-threatening disease, though at times a combination of medications may be required to control the flare up of the disease. According to the National Institute for Health and Care Excellence, people who suffer from psoriatic arthritis have a life expectancy that is three years lower compared to others. It may also be seen as a 60 per cent increase in their mortality. Thus, these people are at risk of dying at an age earlier than the average population.

Based on the research it was found that patients with psoriatic arthritis generally have a vast impact on lowering the health-related quality of life. It was found to be due to a decline in physical status, functions and an increased risk of mortality. Psoriatic arthritis as time progresses leads to complications like involvement of the heart, eyes, skin, lungs or the gut. These factors are an added risk for increasing the mortality. The added joint pain and inflammation leads to immobility, which has a dual effect on the overall wellness of the patient. The negative aspects such as unhappiness, depression and mood swings about their functional disability may lead to the worsening of their performance. Researchers have shown that an increase in stress has been found to be directly related to progression of the disease, though there are always conflicting views still going on about this.

Psoriatic arthritis is a disease that can have a waxing and waning pattern. The person may be all right for a long time without any flare-ups or they may have flare-ups on and off with shorter symptom-free intervals. With adequate and aggressive treatment with medications, exercise and physiotherapy, excellent outcomes can be achieved. The main key is to start the therapy as soon as the disease has been diagnosed. More and more medications that are extremely potent and effective have been produced to deal with unresponsive patients or those who have not been successfully treated with other conventional medications. As there is no prevention of psoriatic arthritis, it is advised to seek medical opinion as soon as possible. Therefore the earlier the treatment is begun when the pain is minimal, the lesser is the joint damage and better results are observed. People who are overweight can benefit from asking their doctors about weight-lowering exercises and treatment so as to lower the disease progression. It may help in reducing the stress on the joints of the body due to the extra weight. Others may find cod liver oil beneficial for them as it helps in reducing inflammation in the body, therefore it may be worth a try. Alcohol consumption is another factor that needs to be tapered so as to lessen the inflammation in the body. Males or females of childbearing ages who are planning to start a family must consult their doctor regarding their disease. The reason is, their treatment may need to be changed or their dose adjusted according to their body requirements. Women of childbearing ages may need extra childcare during their pregnancies. There may be no flare-ups during pregnancy but the disease may progress faster after childbirth. So, it is important for would-be mothers to seek care before and after their pregnancy to deal with the pregnancy-related outcomes of psoriatic arthritis. Similarly, a person may need to do work adjustments so as to have a normal work or career life.

Cognitive behavioural therapy and psychotherapy have been advised for people who have not seen any improvement with counselling. For many years, these therapies have proved useful in controlling the negative effects related to psoriatic arthritis. Meanwhile, other people have found support groups to be helpful in fighting off the disease, especially during flare-ups. There is no limitation of activities that have been suggested to be avoided in psoriatic arthritis. Any activity that was enjoyed previously can be carried out easily as long as there is no increase in joint damage. Persons with psoriatic arthritis may need emotional help from their family or friends to help in understanding the disease during the times of frustration and flare-ups. It may seem hard to deal with their anger or mood swings during those times but helping them out of it is as important as is taking medications.

Psoriatic Arthritis & Vitamin D

Treatment with vitamin D may help people with psoriatic arthritis as shown in some research studies. Some researchers have postulated that modifying the causative agent in the progression of psoriatic arthritis, especially the immune system to make the genetics better, improves the efficacy of medical treatments.

The long-term prognosis for the management of psoriatic arthritis is good, especially with the on-going researches and medications. The goal is to be compliant with medications and treatment so as to achieve maximum benefits along with changes in the mind set with a positive approach towards the disease.

Chapter 8: Current and Potential Applications of Pharmacogenetics & Pharmacogenomics

Apart from NSAIDs and steroid therapy, there are other drugs on the market that can help to manage the pain and swelling of joints in patients with psoriatic arthritis. These treatments have undergone extensive research and their credibility may be questioned based on the fact that there are still many clinical trials going on. The future for patients with psoriatic arthritis is looking bright in terms of newer medications and treatments on the market. At the beginning of the twentieth century there were no clear treatments as to how the disease can be controlled. But now it seems that psoriatic arthritis has been recognised as a special entity and more research has been conducted for its treatment.

It is mandatory to identify patients with a greater risk of treatment toxicity or non-response prior to starting the treatment. With the discovery of predictive markers of treatment response, it would be very helpful in determining the response to therapies. Thus the role of pharmacogenomics is increasingly important in healthcare so as to reach an ultimate goal for the treatment of psoriatic arthritis. Such a goal is important to help safely individualise patients and minimise the unnecessary expenditure. The treatment can therefore be tailored and monitored according to each individual patient and not treated conventionally.

To be able to differentiate the mechanism, the effects of pharmacogenomics and pharmacogenetics of various drugs including the methotrexate, cyclosporine, TNF- alpha inhibitors, eflizumab, alefacept and narrow band UVB phototherapy is critically vital. Psoriatic arthritis is a complex disease where there is a combination of many factors that play an equally important role in disease progression and modification. The environment, genetics and clinical influences are known to help modify and control disease progression. Therefore, to achieve maximum effect from treatments it is necessary to personalise the management of the disease. The growing fields of research are helpful in providing a safer and more effective treatment regimen for psoriatic arthritis.

The pathogenesis of psoriatic arthritis is not fully understood but environmental factors and genetics have played important roles leading to a regulation of both human immunity and other specific immunity. There was seen to be a strong correlation in the family studies and well as a factor known as human leukocyte antigen that is thought to increase the immune-related response in the body. One amongst many other genes such as the HLA Cw-6 has shown significant association with the development of psoriatic arthritis. The disease onset with the age of 40 has been strongly linked to a higher frequency of gene HLA –Cw6. This has a bond with the occurrence of a positive family history of psoriatic arthritis. Understanding of the pharmacogenomic markers helps in treating psoriatic arthritis in a better way. The study of relations of DNA and RNA characteristics is related to the drug response of the patient. **Pharmacogenetics is therefore related to the study of relationships between individual gene variations and drug responses.** Variation in the genetic makeup affects the drug metabolising enzymes, drug transporters and drug target sites, hence it is responsible for drug interactions. The use of pharmacogenetic markers is now being applied directly to help modulate immune related responses and chemotherapy in many diseases. In psoriatic arthritis, its use is taking place with the evaluation of the genes responsible for drug metabolising enzymes and genes that are susceptible for psoriasis.

In science, **pharmacogenomics is basically the application of pharmacogenetics to examine the influences of genetic variation correlating to the drug responses**. The efficacy of the drug or its toxicity related to the genetic response is vital in determining the course of psoriatic arthritis. It has been noticed that the treatment response to psoriatic arthritis has not been constant, as patients frequently lose their response to drugs over time or sometimes they fail to respond to treatments that were successfully used on others. Sometimes the second therapy response has shown absolutely no results that were proven to be quiet effective in the beginning of the disease. Changes in the RNA and DNA factors can help to achieve the much-desired responses to treatment, making it an easier option to deal with psoriatic arthritis, also acquiring good results with previous non-responders to treatment.

Methotrexate has been used for controlling the symptoms of psoriatic arthritis for more than 50 years now. It has a potent effect on the immune system and it modulates the immunity by suppressing the response. hence known for its anti-inflammatory actions. The studies conducted to assess the effect of methotrexate and its toxic results showed that genetics do play a major role in the variability of its efficacy and toxicity. But no conclusive studies have been presented as a sure thing for making methotrexate an obsolete drug for the treatment of psoriatic arthritis.

Cyclosporine is another drug that has been successfully used to treat moderate to severe cases of psoriatic arthritis. Cyclosporine has a limited window for use due to its major side effects like hypertension, hyperlipidaemia and other neurologic effect. Cyclosporine is also lacking in pharmacogenetic studies in patients with psoriatic arthritis. It is known for its effect on the cells that enhance inflammatory mediators within the body.

A vitamin A derivative, Acitretin, has been in use for psoriatic arthritis since the year 1980. With a mechanism similar to cyclosporine, it down regulates the inflammatory cells, decreasing the inflammation of the joints. The VEGF gene has been associated with an enhanced expression of psoriatic arthritis in susceptible people. Therefore, such a retinoid as Acitretin blocks the VEGF gene in order to suppress inflammatory responses.

TNF-alpha Inhibitors are the revolutionary drugs in the treatment of psoriasis and psoriatic arthritis. Being an expensive medication on the market, their affordability can be an issue with the average population. The side effects are notorious as well due to its pharmacological action as being the strongest drug. The therapy response is still variable, which raises a question about its efficacy. Some of the known TNF-alpha inhibitors are Infliximab and adalimumab, whereas the etanercept is a recombinant human TNF-alpha receptor-acting drug. Pharmacogenetic studies are lacking in support for the use of these TNF-alpha inhibitors. However, using these TNF-alpha inhibitor studies suggesting its use for rheumatoid arthritis has been conflicting so far. Studies which have a HLA-Cw6 gene have not shown any association with response to treatment with these TNF-alpha inhibitors.

Alefacept is a human fusion protein related to antibodies and is biologic therapy approved in the year 2003 for its use in psoriasis. It was well known for having a significant and prolonged period of remission for the duration of approximately 7-8 months, mainly after a single course of 12 weeks. Hence this feature made it an ideal drug for pharmacogenomic studies. The study consisted of responders and non-responders to alefacept related to gene expression. Alefacept down regulated several genes related to the immunity like the T cells and natural killer cells in responders. While as in the non-responders subjects there was an over-expression of other immune-related cells. Hence, it was concluded that there are some genes that are over-expressed in the non-responders which made it difficult for them to respond better to alefacept therapy.

Anti IL12-23 antibodies are still under investigation regarding their action on psoriatic arthritis patients. They have been linked strongly with the over-expression in genetic makeup, therefore causing plaque formation and lesions in various joints.

Phototherapy with Narrowband UVB is extremely beneficial and cost-effective in psoriatic arthritis patients. Before starting the therapy, all patients should undergo excessive examination and a thorough history should be obtained from them. The key factor is consistency and compliance with a session usually three times weekly. This regimen, though being tremendously beneficial, has its own down side; shortage of time, work commitments and day to day busy life. The response of patients to Narrowband UVB would help to determine such therapies that can be targeted directly at psoriatic arthritis patients. In due time, this treatment will also help to limit the period of remissions by affecting the vitamin D status. So it is safe to say that VDR gene expression that is linked to vitamin D can be determined by how strongly the patient responds to Narrowband UVB therapy. In pregnant patients as well, UVB light therapy is considered to be safe. Care must be taken, especially with patients undergoing chronic sessions of UVB therapy and appropriate eye protection should be worn to avoid any injury to the eyes. UVA light therapy is more effective than UVB light but it has a greater risk of toxicity and carcinogenic effects.

Psoriatic arthritis being a chronic and life-long disease has been frequently treated using combination therapies. In moderate to severe cases, a combination of alefacept or efalizumab and narrowband UVB phototherapy has been successfully used.

Vitamin D analogues, usually when used topically, have known to improve psoriatic arthritis. The response is nothing dramatic but it has helped to minimise the symptoms related to pain, joint inflammation and stiffness. The VDR gene is held responsible for the expression of psoriatic plaques that end up damaging the joints.

Lastly, coal tar preparations have been used for over 100 years as a topical remedy for psoriatic arthritis. Although the toxic effects related to coal tar preparations cannot be denied, it still carries a high risk for causing mutant-like changes in the genetic structure.

Chapter 9: Surgery in Psoriatic Arthritis

In today's time, there is so much knowledge about the joint inflammation and pain related to psoriatic arthritis that it has led to the discovery of newer medications. Though psoriatic arthritis has been proved to have no cure, the damage can be controlled and minimised by the constant use of medications.

Some people suffering from psoriatic arthritis have a relatively serious condition and it requires them to use a combination of medications in order to control their symptoms and prevent further joint damage. Therefore, doctors all over the world consider psoriatic arthritis to be a treatable disease rather than a curable one.

The medications used to treat psoriatic arthritis work differently on different people. The strongest medications are considered as the last option due to their serious side effects on the body. Other options like splints or braces have been proved to be helpful in lessening the joint damage, controlling the pain and joint stiffness.

Doctors recommend surgery when there is massive joint damage due to psoriatic arthritis. Due to the limitation of surgical options, only joint replacement has been suggested for serious conditions. In this surgery, the joint is replaced by an artificial joint. Of course, there can be a relapse or worsening of the conditions after replacement but that has been seen rarely.

The team of doctors including the surgeons, rheumatologists, dermatologists and other physicians can help determine whether the results of surgery would be beneficial for the patient. After the surgery is done the patient needs to be on immune-suppressing drugs to avoid the flare-up of the immunity against the artificially placed joints. The post-surgical treatment is as important as any other decision in tackling psoriatic arthritis. Especially in people who suffer from diabetes mellitus, cardiovascular or other metabolic diseases, it becomes difficult to handle these co-morbidities all at the same time. In addition, compliance in such patients can be very tricky, as managing more than one medication can be difficult. Hence, surgery is recommended as the only option for very few people when it becomes absolutely necessary.

Professional Advice: Surgery is mostly considered as a last treatment option or under inevitably severe conditions. However, there are some individuals who avoid surgical operations and opt for alternative options on a priority basis. The following diet section can hugely help such individuals to cope with their PA naturally without any surgeries.

Chapter 10: Psoriatic Arthritis & The Need Of A Specific Diet

The future can be set today. I can decide today how I want to end up tomorrow. I can design my destiny. Similarly, food choices that we make in the present can decide what kind of health we want to have in the future. The *National Institute on Aging* (associated with U.S Department of Health & Services) states that the top ten most life-threatening chronic illnesses are directly associated with either malnutrition or unhealthy eating habits. Balanced nutritional support is mandatory to maintain health and to survive. Water, fats, minerals, vitamins and proteins are five main types of nutrients we must take in. Nevertheless, this is not enough and we have to consume these basic nutrients in calculated proportions to maintain a balance. Sustaining this balance over a long period of time is crucial for the protection against illnesses, physical and mental disorders and to meet the most demanding physical challenges.

Similarly, diet plays an equally critical role for Psoriatic Arthritis patients. Disturbing feelings of pain, discomfort, agony, infliction and annoyance related to Psoriatic Arthritis can be treated or limited to a certain extent with a properly planned diet.

Unhealthy Food Consumption & Chronic Illnesses:

Obesity is one of the top health concerns around the globe. Obesity can lead to several chronic illnesses, especially diabetes, cardiovascular disorders (like stroke, high cholesterol level and hypertension), infertility, back-pain and gallstones.

Obviously, obesity is directly related to bad eating. There are certain food items that contribute to being overweight. It is scientifically established that obesity is a health hazard that leads to countless disorders. Sometimes, obesity-induced health problems can be very difficult to diagnose and it takes a lot of time for a physician to actually prescribe the right treatment. Situations this critical and confusing simply imply that every individual has to be very circumspect of his/her daily food choices.

Why A Special Diet for Psoriatic Arthritis?

After years of professional practice, I can articulate that most patients had bad selection of food on regular basis. The unhealthy choice of food can make it even more difficult to cope with any stressful conditions of Psoriatic Arthritis. A lot of work has been done in the field of dietary patterns by nutritionists to ensure the betterment of Psoriatic Arthritis patients. Evolution in the field of "Nutritional Science" has allowed special diets to be devised under anti-inflammatory diet recommendations to help miserable patients. I have added recipes that are delicious to eat and equally healthy. I have selected these recipes from authentic and reliable sources after years of research. I have mentioned nutritional information for each recipe for the readers. You can also use this information to calculate your calorie and nutritional intake on a daily basis. Most of my patients have already benefited from these recipes. Now, I want it to spread to a broader horizon where every one of you can use this book to your advantage.

Primary Healthcare & Its Significance:

The World Health Organization (WHO) started a Primary Health Care (PHC) program under the concept of "Health for all" back in 1978, at Alma Ata, Kazakhstan. The concept was to initiate a program for health contributed to by health institutions, healthcare professionals, doctors, scientific researchers, pharmacological experts, civil society organisations, governments and grassroots organisations. The idea was to eradicate health-related inequalities in all countries around the globe. The point of mentioning *"Primary health Care"* at this point is to enlighten and appreciate the efforts of "WHO" that is thriving to secure health standards everywhere.

What does Special Diet mean for Psoriatic Arthritis?

Every 'Psoriatic Arthritis' patient will come across multiple coping and recovery options and dietary suggestions. However, most health professionals consider an anti-inflammation diet as their number one option to ensure healing and optimal health for Psoriatic Arthritis patients.

Dr. Dickson Thom from the National College of Naturopathic Medicine (NCNM) is one diet expert along with many others who teaches his students about the amazing benefits of the anti-inflammation diet. The diet is termed anti-inflammatory because it excludes all foods that are allergenic in nature and can potentially promote inflammation. An anti-inflammatory diet also eliminates different types of antibiotic residues, hormones and pesticides, processed foods, sugars, toxins, hydrogenated oils and most difficult to digest substances. It is mostly known to include whole foods, vegetables, fruits and foods that are easier to digest. Foods that are known to improve metabolism are also termed as anti-inflammatory foods.

Most individuals and families find it hard to shift to an anti-inflammation diet straight away. The transaction could be slow and gradual in order to adopt dietary habits completely. Timely and healthy changes in dietary habits are also important to ensure reduced chances of future chronic diseases.

Psoriatic Arthritis & Inflammation
To establish a comprehensive understanding of the relation between Psoriatic Arthritis and inflammation there are multiple aspects of the disease to consider, along with the role of inflammation on overall health.

Connection between Inflammation & Chronic Illnesses

The Journal of the American Medical Association and multiple other research sources have supported the possibility of a surprising link between chronic illnesses and chronic inflammation. Chronic illnesses that are included in this category are heart diseases (all disorders related to cardiovascular system), diabetes (especially a risk factor for type-2 diabetes), chronic pain (most common is fibromyalgia) and insomnia.

Beside several health complications, the best news for readers is that the reduction of inflammation through dietary changes can heal damaged tissues, improve sleep patterns and eliminate pain.

Psoriatic Arthritis and Self-Medication

Self-medication is very common in all pain-related disorders. We have several medications used for treating different symptoms of psoriatic arthritis and methotrexate is the most common generic. The drug class named NSAIDs possesses several side effects if used over a long period. However, we will only mention a few side effects of methotrexate (anti-rheumatic agent, immunosuppressive agents) in a list.

FDA Warnings – Methotrexate: - Immunisations,vaccinations, lung disease, intestinal diseases, chickenpox, -alcohol, allergy, kidney disease, liver disease, sensitivity to sun, avoid touching eyes, contraceptive measures, pregnancy, and lactation.

Adverse Reactions or Side Effects:

Generally known Common Side-Effects:

- Nausea, - Vomiting,

- Fever, - Erythema,

- Cough, - Ocular irritation,

- Desquamation,

Generally known Serious Side Effects:

- Nuchal rigidity, - Myelosuppression,

- Coma, - Chemical arachnoiditis,

- Motor paralysis of extremities,

- Cranial nerve palsy, - Dementia, - Nephrotoxicity,

- GI mucositis, - Seizures, - Eelvated hepatic enzymes,

- Pleuritis, - Motor paralysis of extremities,

41

- Pneumonitis, and - Vasculitis.

Psoriatic Arthritis & Food Intolerances:

The human digestive system is unique and demands a calculated approach. A balanced nutritional diet is the only way to a healthy body. Our digestive system is linked to nearly all major organs in the sense that any complications regarding the digestive system can lead to several other health problems. Now, it is very important for us to implement positive dietary and lifestyle changes. A balanced diet with regular exercise can do wonders. A combination of a professionally designed exercise program and healthy diet can guarantee optimal health goals.

We know that specific guidelines can be associated with every diet plan. However, every diet has only one target and that is to achieve long-lasting health. Fighting mild and chronic illnesses through dietary support is one significant tool in every diet. Obviously, a psoriatic arthritis diet (anti-inflammatory diet) is also designed on similar grounds. Additionally, one major factor of anti-inflammatory diet is to eliminate food intolerances. Recent evolution in our food choices has increased the consumption of intolerable agents enormously. American fast food is a prime example of this not-so-good evolution.

Our immune system cannot tolerate certain food proteins. When such food is consumed, our immune system can release histamines as a response. Histamine releases can result in the following responses:

- Watery eyes, runny nose, hives, diarrhoea, abdominal cramping, anaphylaxis and an elevated level of throat mucous.

Foods to Avoid in Psoriatic Arthritis

Here is a list of foods that you should avoid if you are suffering from Psoriatic arthritis.

- Wheat products,

- Dairy products,

- Potatoes,

- Tomatoes,

- Corn,

- Sugar,

- Citrus fruits,

- Pork,

- Commercial (nonorganic) eggs,

- Shellfish,

- Peanuts

- Coffee,

- Alcohol,

- Juice,

- Caffeinated teas,

- Soda,

- Foods containing hydrogenated oils,

- Processed foods,

- Fried foods.

Symptoms of Food Allergies/Intolerances

Foods allergens can cause several symptoms to appear. Here is a list of potential symptoms:

- Headaches,

- Constant clearing of the throat,

- Mucous in the throat,

- Abdominal complaints

- Bloating or cramping,

- Irritable bowel syndrome,

- Irritable bowel disease,

- Aphthous (mouth) ulcers,

- Sinusitis (inflammation of the sinus cavities),

- Runny nose and/or congestion,

- Fatigue,

- Migraines,

- Arthritis,

 - Asthma,

- Eczema,

- Otitis media (ear infection),

- Psoriasis,

- Most skin complaints,

- Acne,

- Chronic cough,

- Chronic allergies to pollens and moulds.

Chapter 11: Psoriatic Arthritis Special Diet

We have already talked about the influence and characteristics of an anti-inflammatory diet. This chapter will explain how we should follow the anti-inflammation diet. First, we need to realise the need of basic constituents to improve basic food intake.

Consumption of Macronutrient in %age for Optimal Health		
1.	Carbohydrate (mostly complex carbohydrates)	40–60 per cent (of total calories)
2.	Fat (balanced essential fatty acids)	20–30 per cent (of total calories)
3.	Protein	20–30 per cent (of total calories)

People all around the world eat a low calorie and low-fat diet to lose weight and to fight inflammation and joint pain. It is true that low-calorie and low fat diets are known to drop fats quickly. However, in the long term, both these styles of eating can result in weight regain. The human body has its own built-in mechanism to maintain its weight. A specific body weight that lasts over a certain period of time is often set as a parameter by our internal mechanism. We can drop unwanted calories in a short duration but it will not be permanent. Whenever we shift to a regular diet, our internal mechanism will store energy to regain weight that was set as a standard parameter. So, instead of restricting your calorie-intake, the better option is to eat the right foods. Eating the right foods that are nutritious and contain fat-burning agents is a better choice for permanent weight-loss, anti-inflammation and optimal health.

The Best Food Choices for Psoriatic Arthritis

The right choice of food can be influential to cope with psoriatic arthritis. In the previous chapter, we have mentioned the foods that you should avoid. Now, note down the following foods choices that will certainly imply positive impact on your illness:

- Filtered water,

- Fruits and vegetables,

- Turmeric, ginger and garlic,

- All nuts and seeds (except peanuts),

- Flaxseed oil, olive oil or vegetable oil,

- Pineapple (contains bromelain to reduce inflammation),

- Essential fatty acids found in fish and fish oils (like halibut, salmon, mackerel, tuna and sardines),

- Organic foods (with less toxic chemicals, colourings and food additives),

- Antioxidants (beneficial vitamins and minerals like iron, zinc, copper, selenium, calcium, vitamin-A, vitamin-C, vitamin-D and folic acid).

Here is a detailed table of the best food choices:

#	Food Category	Healthy Food Choices	Unhealthy Food Choices
1.	**Spices & herbs**	All edible herbs and spices are allowed to enhance the colour & flavour of your food	
2.	**Grains** *(Ideally 1–2 cups/day)*	Barley, buckwheat, Amaranth, spelt, millet, oatmeal, brown rice, rye, quinoa, basmati rice & rice crackers	All kind of wheat products (like whole-wheat flour, breads, white flour, cereals & pasta-made from wheat
3.	**Legumes** *(Soak legumes well before cooking)*	Garbanzo beans, split peas, lentils, kidney beans, pinto beans, black beans, mung beans, fermented soybeans (tempeh or miso) & adzuki beans	Tofu
4.	**Seafood** *(Deep-sea, cold-water & wild)*	Cod, wild salmon, haddock, tuna, trout, halibut, mackerel, sardines, & summer flounder	Shrimp, shellfish, lobster, clams, crab & mussels
5.	**Meat** *(best in small quantity with every meal to regulate*	Wild game, venison, organic chicken, organic turkey, organic lamb and	Pork

	blood sugar and energy levels)	buffalo.	
6.	**Fruits** *(Limit to 1–2 servings/day)*	Bananas, figs, prunes, pineapples, pomegranates, cherries, grapes, pears, apples, blueberries, cranberries, papayas, apricots, blackberries, raspberries, kiwis, peaches, plums, melons, strawberries, cantaloupe & rhubarb.	
7.	**Vegetables:**	Yams, sweet Potatoes, green peas, winter squash, carrots, artichokes, parsnips, cucumber, endive, lettuce, cauliflower, celery, Swiss chard, beet greens, broccoli, red and green cabbage, asparagus, beansprouts, chives, collards, eggplant, kale, kohlrabi, leeks, onion, string beans, beets, bokchoy, Brussels sprouts, parsley, red pepper, pumpkin, turnips, rutabagas &zucchini	Tomatoes & potatoes
8.	**Eggs & dairy products**	Organic eggs	Most Dairy products (like cheese and yogurt) &

			commercial eggs
9.	*Butter & oils (make spread by using 1- pound organic butter with 1 cup extra-virgin olive oil)*	Small amount of organic butter, olive oil for cooking, nut or seed oils for salads and olive oil for cooking	Trans fats, hydrogenated oils, partially hydrogenated oils
10.	*Sweetener s(allowed occasionally)*	Raw honey, agave syrup, pure maple syrup, brown rice syrup & stevia	Sugar &NutraSweet
11	*Nuts & seeds (eat raw or add grinded in salads, cereals, steamed vegetables & cooked Grains)*	Sesame, sunflower seeds, Flax, pumpkin, most nuts & nut butters	Peanuts & peanut butter
12	*Beverages*	Herbal teas, limited quantities of rice-milk, oat-milk, Almond-milk, or soy milk	Alcohol, energy drinks, soda, coffee, juice & caffeinated teas
13	*Miscellaneous*		Fried foods, processed foods& corn products

Ideal Lifestyle Choices for Psoriatic Arthritis

Processed sweets, prepared meals, fast food and quick blood-sugar fixes (in the form of candy bars) have become an integral part of our fast-paced life in recent times. Above all, our graph of physical activity is continuously declining in comparison to earlier generations. Unhealthy food and an unhealthy lifestyle are a deadly combination and an open invitation to killer diseases. Most diet plans are followed with exercise programs designed to achieve health-specific goals. Exercise is a lifestyle change that is ranked high for Psoriatic and other types of arthritis patients. The intensity and exercise plans can be different but the need of physical activity remains as it is.

Chapter 12: Meals & Recipes

A clear understanding of the need for a specific diet for Psoriatic Arthritis is already established. Another important thing is to realise the influence of antioxidants in human health. We are well aware of the health advantages of micronutrients. However, we must also know that some micronutrients (minerals and vitamins) act as antioxidants, like vitamin-A, vitamin-C, vitamin-E and zinc. Antioxidants play a vital role in reducing oxidative stress by the excretion of toxins and free radicals from the body.

Free-Radical Theory of Aging (FRTA):

The theory simply explains that cell damage over time can result in aging and several health complications. The cells are damaged as a result of oxidative stress. All the atoms or molecules that are unpaired like superoxide (O_2) and melanin can cause cell damage. Antioxidant intake can help in the prevention of this biological process and maintain good health. The following diets and recipes are also rich in foods that contain antioxidants mentioned above.

Weight Loss Advantage:

All the recipes and diets added in this book can also be used as weight loss diets. The main reason behind these diets' dual anticipation is the elimination of food allergens and presence of anti-inflammatory ingredients. I have made sure that not only the patients of Psoriatic Arthritis are benefited by these diets but also the whole family can maintain their weight and health regardless of the age group. Kids, teenagers and the elderly, all can follow these diet recipes to achieve gradual weight loss. The human body is designed to maintain its shape for a certain time period, that's why if we systematically implement weight loss techniques we can achieve permanent weight control.

(1) Beverages& Teas

1. Herbal Vitality Juice:

The ingredients are healthy and sugar free. This is an easy to prepare, ideal fruit juice replacement. The presence of hibiscus makes it visually appealing as well.

Ingredients: - Dried crataegus leaves (½ cup- hawthorn), - honey (according to taste), - dried crataegusberries (hawthorn) ½ cup, - rose hips (½ cup), - 1 medium lemon (zest), - dried peppermint leaves ((½ cup), - hibiscus flowers (dried ¼ cup).

Store all ingredients mixed together in an airtight jar. Ideally, use 1 tablespoon to prepare 1 cup of tea/juice. You should be creative and adventurous to try different flavours and add natural ingredients to suit your taste and health better.

Instructions: Boil 1 cup of water in a kettle. Add lemon zest and dried herbs in it. Heat it for about 10 to 15 minutes until it reaches boiling point. After 15 minutes the drink is ready. You can add honey (for sweet taste). You can serve it either warm or chilled.

Cornell University conducted a study on 200 children that evaluated that kids should consume no more than 6 ounces of sweetened drinks. Sweetened drinks up to 12 ounces on a regular basis can lead to unhealthy weight gain. So, teas and beverages like *"Herbal Vitality Juice"* are good for children's health.

Here are some teas that are easily prepared by boiling water and adding the desired ingredients, then cooked for about 10 to 15 minutes.

2. Sedating Tea:

Ingredients: - Passionflower (one part), - chamomile flowers (two parts), - hypericum (St. John's Wort): one part, - lavender flowers (one part).

3. Ideal Stress Managing Tea:

Ingredients: - linden-flower (2 parts), - lemon balm (1 part), - oat-straw (2 parts), and passion -flower (1 part).

4. High Energy Tea:

Ingredients: - Gotu kola (one part), - Siberian ginseng (one part), - ginkgo biloba (one part), - licorice (one part).

5. Mood Lifting Tea:

Ingredients: - lemon balm (one part), - passionflower (one part), - hypericum (St. John's Wort): one part.

6. Detoxification/Cleansing Tea:

Ingredients: - Pure maple syrup (1 tablespoon), - filtered water (8 to 10 ounces), - cayenne (¼ teaspoon). The quantity of cayenne should be according to your taste.

7. Purifying Tea:

Ingredients: - Burdock root (one part), - liquorice root (two parts), - dandelion root (one part).

8. Digestion Friendly Tea:

Ingredients: - Fennel (one part), - peppermint (two parts), - anise seed (one part), - gingerroot (½ part).

9. Immunity Enhancer Tea:

Ingredients: - Liquorice (one part), - elderberry (two parts), - hyssop (one part), - peppermint (two parts), - Echinacea (two parts), - thyme (one part).

10. Nerve Relaxant Tea:

Ingredients: - Hibiscus flowers (one part), - basil (one part), - peppermint (two parts), - lemon balm (one part), - catnip (one part).

11. Healthy/Smooth Sleep Tea:

Ingredients: - Passionflower (one part), - valerian (optional) (one part), - skullcap (two parts), - chamomile (two parts).

Instructions: All these teas are very easy to prepare and the cooking time is similar to 15 minutes for each tea. The teas are formed to provide soothing and anti-inflammatory effects. You can certainly experiment by swapping a couple of herbs here and there. Honey and lemon zest are two ingredients that you are free to add according to your taste in whichever tea you like. Additionally, these teas are meant to sooth inflammation and these recipes can be used as complementary treatment alongside main medications. However, these diets and recipes should not be considered as a potential replacement for the main medication for Psoriatic Arthritis or any other form of arthritis.

12. Nutritious Almond Milk:

The basic ingredient in this beverage is almond milk, which contains potent fatty acids. Almond milk can be consumed as it is and is easily available at all stores. It is better than cow's milk and contains plant-based fatty acids.

*Detailed nutritional breakup:

Nutritional Value For Each Recipe: Nutritious Almond Milk: Serving Size: 4					
/TOTAL CALORIES	105.3g	/Vitamin-A	0.2RE	Potassium	124mg
/TOTAL FAT	9.2g	/Vitamin-C	0mg	Zinc	0.6mg
/SATURATED FAT	0.7g	/Thiamin (B-1)	0mg	Magnesium	49mg
/CARBO-HYDRATE	3.6g	/Riboflavin (B-2)	0.1mg	Phosphorus	87mg
/FIBER	1.9g	/Vitamin B-12	0µg	Iron	0.7mg
/CHOLESTEROL	0mg	/Vitamin B-6	0mg	Calcium	39mg
/PROTEIN	4g	/Niacin	0.7mg	Vitamin-E	0mg
/SODIUM	5.1mg	/Folate	5.4µg	Vitamin-D	0µg

13. Goodly Sesame Milk:

Goodly sesame milk is a powerful combination of protein and essential nutrients. Rice milk can be added in equal quantity to prepare a scrumptious drink.

Ingredients: - Sesame seeds (one cup), - carob powder (2 teaspoons), - filtered water (3½ cups), - honey (1 tablespoon).

*Detailed nutritional breakup of the recipe:

Nutritional Value For Each Recipe: Goodly Sesame Milk: Serving Size: 4					
/TOTAL CALORIES	121.5g	/Vitamin-A	0.2RE	Potassium	95.8mg
/TOTAL FAT	8.9g	/Vitamin-C	0mg	Zinc	1.4mg
/SATURATED FAT	1.3g	/Thiamin (B-1)	0.1mg	Magnesium	63.9mg
/CARBO-HYDRATE	9.5g	/Riboflavin (B-2)	0mg	Phosphorus	114mg
/FIBER	2.6g	/Vitamin B-12	0µg	Iron	2.7mg
/CHOLESTEROL	0mg	/Vitamin B-6	0.1mg	Calcium	179mg
/PROTEIN	3.2g	/Niacin	0.8mg	Vitamin-E	0mg
/SODIUM	2.6mg	/Folate	17.9µg	Vitamin-D	0µg

Instructions: Soak sesame seeds (one cup) in 3½ cups filtered water overnight. Next morning, rinse and drain them. Use a blender and add carob powder and honey and blend until smooth. Godly sesame milk is ready to sooth your body.

(2) Breakfasts

1. Quick 5-min Breakfast:

This recipe is very easy to prepare. You can use leftover brown rice. We have already suggested some food items you must have in your kitchen. Storing canned and cooked food in advance allows you to prepare meals and breakfast quickly. Seeds, raisins and nuts should be at your disposal 24/7.

Ingredients: - Cooked brown rice (leftover, 1 cup), - chopped walnuts (¼ cup), - sunflower seeds (¼ cup), - rice milk (½ cup), or other alternative milk (½ cup), - cinnamon powder (¼ teaspoon), - raisins (1/8 cup), - carob powder according to taste (¼ teaspoon), - maple syrup (½ teaspoon). Instructions: Mix all the ingredients and heat. Use milk to cover the rice. Warm up to cereal consistency and serve.

*Detailed nutritional breakup of the recipe:

Nutritional Value For Each Recipe: Quick 5-min Breakfast: Serving Size: 6.					
/TOTAL CALORIES	370g	/Vitamin-A	1.7 RE	Potassium	378.6 mg
/TOTAL FAT	20.4g	/Vitamin-C	0.8 mg	Zinc	2.2mg
/SATURATED FAT	2.2g	/Thiamin (B-1)	0.1 mg	Magnesium	142.8 mg
/CARBO-HYDRATE	40.7g	/Riboflavin (B-2)	0.1 mg	Phosphorus	295.3 mg
/FIBER	5.2g	/Vitamin B-12	0.4µg	Iron	2.6 mg
/CHOLESTEROL	0mg	/Vitamin B-6	0mg	Calcium	64mg
/PROTEIN	11g	/Niacin	2.7 mg	Vitamin-E	0.1mg
/SODIUM	28mg	/Folate	66.6µg	Vitamin-D	0µg

2. Powerhouse Tasty Granola:

You can prepare this old dish with new changes at home to make sure that there are no hydrogenated oils and additives present. Most commercial granola available is full of hydrogenated oils and additives.

Ingredients: - Rolled oats (6 cups), - sunflower seeds (1 cup raw, shelled), - sesame seeds (½ cup), - unsweetened coconut (1¼ cups), - almonds (chopped, 1 cup), - organic coconut oil (½ cup), and - honey (½ cup).

Instructions: First, preheat your oven to 325°F. Now, mix all above-mentioned dry ingredients in a bowl. Prepare a liquid sauce using oil and honey in a saucepan. Add this sauce to the dry ingredients and mix them together. Once the mixture is ready, bake it in the oven for 15-20 minutes. Your home cooked granola is ready. You should cook in large quantities to refrigerate it for later use. Ideally, eat with milk or proffered fruit.

*Detailed nutritional breakup of the recipe:

Nutritional Value For Each Recipe: Powerhouse Tasty Granola: Serving Size: 14.					
/TOTAL CALORIES	317.9 g	/Vitamin-A	0.7 RE	Potassium	241.3 mg
/TOTAL FAT	23.4g	/Vitamin-C	0.4 mg	Zinc	102.5 mg
/SATURATED FAT	10.3g	/Thiamin (B-1)	0.4 Mg	Magnesium	210 Mg
/CARBO-HYDRATE	24.3g	/Riboflavin (B-2)	0.1 mg	Phosphorus	0.3mg
/FIBER	4.7g	/Vitamin B-12	0µg	Iron	2.6 mg
/CHOLESTEROL	0mg	/Vitamin B-6	0.2 Mg	Calcium	93.2 mg
/PROTEIN	7.2g	/Niacin	1.1 mg	Vitamin-E	0mg
/SODIUM	3.3 mg	/Folate	36.8 µg	Vitamin-D	0µg

3. Mexican Egg Breakfast:

This is certainly one of the most delicious and nutritious breakfasts for Psoriatic arthritis patients. It is very easy to prepare with some leftover brown rice.

Ingredients: - Cooked brown rice (leftover, 1 cup) - avocado (1 medium, diced), - organic eggs (four), should be cooked the way you like, - black beans (¾ cup-home-cooked), - chilli powder (½ teaspoon), - sea salt (½ teaspoon), - cumin (½ teaspoon), and - paprika (½ teaspoon).

Instructions: Cook beans, rice and seasonings combined at low-medium heat. Prepare eggs separately. Add eggs to the rice once the rice and beans are warm. Add chopped avocado and serve.

*Detailed nutritional breakup of the recipe:

Nutritional Value For Each Recipe: Mexican Egg Breakfast: Serving Size: 4.					
/TOTAL CALORIES	303.7 g	/Vitamin-A	198.5 RE	Potassium	607.8 mg
/TOTAL FAT	16.1g	/Vitamin-C	6.7 Mg	Zinc	1.6mg
/SATURATED FAT	3.4g	/Thiamin (B-1)	0.2 mg	Magnesiu m	53.7 mg
/CARBO-HYDRATE	29.4g	/Riboflavin (B-2)	0.4 mg	Phosphorus	214.3 mg
/FIBER	8.4g	/Vitamin B-12	0.9µg	Iron	2.9 Mg
/CHOLESTEROL	282.0 mg	/Vitamin B-6	0.4 mg	Calcium	84.6m g
/PROTEIN	13.8g	/Niacin	2.2 mg	Vitamin-E	0mg
/SODIUM	734 mg	/Folate	85.1 µg	Vitamin-D	0.9µg

(3) Appetizers

1. Lemon Flavoured Asparagus:

Nutmeg and lemon both add great flavour to dishes along with several nutritional benefits.

Ingredients: - Juice of lemon (1 medium), - 1 pound asparagus (about 2 bunches), - ground cashews (1 tablespoon, for garnish), - sea salt (½ teaspoon), - black pepper (¼ teaspoon), - olive oil (3 tablespoons), - ground nutmeg (¼ teaspoon).

Instructions: Use washed asparagus with both ends cut. Steam the asparagus but make sure it remains crispy from the inside. Now, prepare lemon juice by mixing oil, lemon juice, nutmeg, salt and pepper. Add this mixture to asparagus arranged on a serving dish. Put some ground cashews on the dish before serving.

*Detailed nutritional breakup of the recipe:

Nutritional Value For Each Recipe: Lemon Flavoured Asparagus: Serving Size: 4.					
/TOTAL CALORIES	128.4	/Vitamin-A	62.8 RE	Potassium	257.6 mg
/TOTAL FAT	11.3g	/Vitamin-C	10.7 mg	Zinc	0.7mg
/SATURATED FAT	1.7g	/Thiamin (B-1)	0.2mg	Magnesium	22.7 mg
/CARBO-HYDRATE	6.2g	/Riboflavin (B-2)	0.2mg	Phosphorus	70.7 mg
/FIBER	2.6g	/Vitamin B-12	0µg	Iron	2.7mg
/CHOLESTEROL	0.0mg	/Vitamin B-6	0.1mg	Calcium	30.1 mg
/PROTEIN	2.9g	/Niacin	1.1mg	Vitamin-E	0mg
/SODIUM	293mg	/Folate	53.2µg	Vitamin-D	0µg

2. Healthy Mexican Guacamole:

It is a full of taste and very easy to make Mexican dish. This dish is full of micronutrients like vitamin-A, foliate, vitamin-c, potassium, magnesium, calcium and phosphorus.

Ingredients: -

Avocados (three, ripe), - garlic cloves (two, minced), - small onion (½ –1, minced-optional), - lemon juice (2 tablespoons), - fresh cilantro (2–3 tablespoons, minced-optional), - pepper (according to taste), - wheat-free tamari (1 teaspoon), - sea salt (according to taste). Suggestions: You can try cottage cheese, 1/4 cup of salsa and sour cream to add flavour to your dish.

Instructions: Put mashed avocados in a mixing bowl and add lemon juice to it. Put the remaining ingredients in their proposed proportions and mix well. Allow the mixture to jolt together for at least half an hour for improved taste.

*Detailed nutritional breakup of the recipe:

Nutritional Value For Each Recipe: Healthy Mexican Guacamole: Serving Size: 6.					
/TOTAL CALORIES	145.0	/Vitamin-A	51.8 RE	Potassium	442.4 mg
/TOTAL FAT	13.1g	/Vitamin-C	10.1 mg	Zinc	0.6mg
/SATURATED FAT	1.8g	/Thiamin (B-1)	0.1 mg	Magnesium	25.5 mg
/CARBO-HYDRATE	8.2g	/Riboflavin (B-2)	0.1 mg	Phosphorus	48.9 mg
/FIBER	5.8g	/Vitamin B-12	0.0µg	Iron	0.6 mg
/CHOLESTEROL	0.0mg	/Vitamin B-6	0.3 mg	Calcium	13.4 mg
/PROTEIN	1.8g	/Niacin	1.7 mg	Vitamin-E	1.1mg
/SODIUM	62.9 mg	/Folate	76.3 µg	Vitamin-D	0.0µg

(4) Side Dishes

1. Rice with Herbal Blend:

Remember to replace your daily intake of white rice with brown rice due to low glycaemic index. This can be a healthy, soothing dish for psoriatic arthritis patients, as well as a fun dish for guests.

However, diabetic patients should not make this dish because of the higher percentage of carbohydrates and sugar content.

Ingredients: - Filtered water (2 cups), - basmati rice (1 cup), - poppy seeds (1½ teaspoons), - lemon juice (2 teaspoons, fresh), - olive oil (6 teaspoons), or olive oil/butter mixture (6 teaspoons), - lemon wedges (for garnish), and - sea salt (½ teaspoon, optional).

Instructions: Very simple to cook; just like boiling plain rice. Add all ingredients and set to boil.

*Detailed nutritional breakup of the recipe:

Nutritional Value For Each Recipe: Rice with Herbal Blend: Serving Size: 6.					
/TOTAL CALORIES	150.6	/Vitamin-A	0.0 RE	Potassium	7.0mg
/TOTAL FAT	4.8g	/Vitamin-C	0.8 Mg	Zinc	0.1mg
/SATURATED FAT	0.7g	/Thiamin (B-1)	0.0mg	Magnesium	2.4 mg
/CARBO-HYDRATE	24.3g	/Riboflavin (B-2)	0.0mg	Phosphorus	6.0 mg
/FIBER	0.4g	/Vitamin B-12	0µg	Iron	0.3mg
/CHOLESTEROL	0.0mg	/Vitamin B-6	0.0mg	Calcium	10.3 mg
/PROTEIN	2.9g	/Niacin	0mg	Vitamin-E	0mg
/SODIUM	0.3mg	/Folate	1.6µg	Vitamin-D	0µg

2. Yummy Salad Rolls:

These rolls are very famous in Vietnamese and Thai cuisine.

Ingredients: - Round rice paper (10 sheets), - rice noodles, use small package (cooked and rinsed), - cilantro (as minced or whole) - one bunch with stems removed, - tofu (½ pound cut into small strips), - carrots (2 medium, also cut into small strips), - cucumber (take half cut lengthwise), and - green leaf lettuce (take small amount and shredded).

Instructions: Another easy recipe. First of all, cut and mix all the ingredients as stated. Make rolls by filling this mixture in sheets (rice paper). Place a pan on the stove to fry the rolls. Put little olive oil in the pan and cook the rolls to light brown. Tasty and yummy salad rolls are ready to eat.

This dish is a perfect source of potassium, phosphorus, calcium and vitamin-A, yet has a very limited quantity of fats and cholesterol. Ideal for heart patients and people having nutritional deficiencies of potassium, vitamin-A and calcium.

*Detailed nutritional breakup of the recipe:

Nutritional Value For Each Recipe:					
Yummy-tasty Salad Rolls::Serving Size: 10.					
/TOTAL CALORIES	143.8	/Vitamin-A	363.2 RE	Potassium	227.8 mg
/TOTAL FAT	6.9g	/Vitamin-C	1.8 mg	Zinc	1.1mg
/SATURATED FAT	1.0g	/Thiamin (B-1)	0.1 mg	Magnesium	43.2 mg
/CARBO-HYDRATE	11.4g	/Riboflavin (B-2)	0.1 mg	Phosphorus	138 Mg
/FIBER	2.2g	/Vitamin B-12	0µg	Iron	2.0mg
/CHOLESTEROL	0.0mg	/Vitamin B-6	0.1 mg	Calcium	473.6 mg
/PROTEIN	11.7g	/Niacin	0.4 mg	Vitamin-E	0mg
/SODIUM	129.0 mg	/Folate	24.2 µg	Vitamin-D	0µg

3. Vegetables Cooked in Steam:

Psoriatic arthritis patients must be aware of the term bento. It is a famous anti-inflammatory style of food in Japan. It is a classical blend of anti-inflammatory sauce, brown rice and various steamed vegetables like zucchini, summer squash, peas, parsnips, carrots, artichokes, turnips, winter squash, garlic, cabbage, sweet peppers, beets, asparagus, cauliflower, broccoli tips, onions, green beans, sweet potatoes, celery, broccoli stalks and mushrooms. Pick your favourite vegetables and cut them into pieces. Place them in a steamer to cook until desired. Electric steamers are ideal to use with exact timers available to you.

(5) Tortillas & Muffins

1. Flour-Rice Muffin:

A very common problem with most of the anti-inflammatory and other weight loss diets is that most of them lack taste. That is why mostly people fail to follow such diets. I must ask readers to try this recipe and they will not be disappointed.

Ingredients: - Rice flour (two cups), - dry yeast granules (four teaspoons), - warm water (½ cup), - honey (2 teaspoons plus ¼ cup), - tapioca flour (2 cups), - vinegar (1 teaspoon), - xanthan gum (4 teaspoons), - it is easily available in health-food stores, - sea salt (1½ teaspoons), - soy milk (1¼ cups), - organic eggs (three, gently beaten), and - melted organic butter (4 tablespoons).

*Detailed nutritional breakup of the recipe:

Nutritional Value For Each Recipe:					
Flour-Rice Muffin: Serving Size: 10-12 muffins.					
/TOTAL CALORIES	533.9	/Vitamin-A	95.1 RE	Potassium	236.7 mg
/TOTAL FAT	12.1 g	/Vitamin-C	56.1 mg	Zinc	1.1mg
/SATURATED FAT	6.0g	/Thiamin (B-1)	0.2 mg	Magnesium	37.9 mg
/CARBO-HYDRATE	96.7g	/Riboflavin (B-2)	0.3 mg	Phosphorus	180.7 mg
/FIBER	3.5g	/Vitamin B-12	0.3 µg	Iron	2.0mg
/CHOLESTEROL	126.1 mg	/Vitamin B-6	0.3 mg	Calcium	56.1 mg
/PROTEIN	10.2g	/Niacin	2.9 mg	Vitamin-E	0mg

/SODIUM	740.1 mg	/Folate	84.3 µg	Vitamin-D	0.5µg

2. Sweet Tasty Muffins:

These muffins are so tasty and sweet that you can even serve them as dessert. Kids will love these muffins due to the added flavour of honey.

Ingredients: - Organic butter (3 tablespoons, melted), - baking powder (1 teaspoon), - soda (½ teaspoon), - milk substitute (½ cup, you can use soy milk or water), - honey (½ cup), - organic egg (one), - oat flour (2 cups), - sea salt (½ teaspoon), - millet (1 cup, uncooked), and - guar gum (½ teaspoon).

Instructions for both muffin recipes: Put all wet food items in a bowl and mix them well. Add dry ingredients gradually in that mixture. Now put millet at the end and stir again.

Now pour the mixture into muffin tin and bake it in preheated oven at 375ºF for about 18 to 20 minutes. It will allow you to make 12 regular muffins.

*Detailed nutritional breakup of the recipe:

Nutritional Value For Each Recipe:					
Sweet Tasty Muffins: Serving Size: 12 muffins.					
/TOTAL CALORIES	210.1	/Vitamin-A	34.0 RE	Potassium	126.5 mg
/TOTAL FAT	5.6 g	/Vitamin-C	0.1 mg	Zinc	1.0mg
/SATURATED FAT	2.3g	/Thiamin (B-1)	0.2 mg	Magnesium	46.6 mg
/CARBO-HYDRATE	35.4g	/Riboflavin (B-2)	0.1 mg	Phosphorus	146.4 mg
/FIBER	2.7g	/Vitamin B-12	0.1 µg	Iron	1.4mg
/CHOLESTEROL	26.5 mg	/Vitamin B-6	0.1 mg	Calcium	41.1 mg
/PROTEIN	5.3g	/Niacin	1.1	Vitamin-E	0.1mg

/SODIUM	233.2 mg	/Folate	mg 23.5 µg	Vitamin-D	0.1µg

(6) Entrées

1. Chicken with Coconut & Almond:

A very healthy, tasty and soothing dish that you can serve both warm and cold. You can also replace rice with any grains of your choice. Replacing rice with other grains will allow the inclusion of more nutrition intake.

Ingredients: - Olive oil (2 teaspoons), - green onions chopped (only to use their white part), - garlic cloves (four, minced), - smooth almond butter (½ cup), - light coconut milk (1 cup), - fresh lemon juice (2 tablespoons), - fish sauce (1 tablespoon), - water (½ cup), - boneless and skinless organic chicken breasts cut in cubes (take 2–3 pieces that will be about 1½ pounds meat), - wheat-free tamari (2 tablespoons), - broccoli chopped (2 heads, including the stalk), - thin rice noodles (½ pound) (you can see cooking instructions for noodles on the packet), - for garnish use dried cranberries (¼ cup), - for garnish also use roasted nuts (¼ cup).

How to cook: Cook garlic and onions in olive oil until light brown. Then, blend these onions and garlic along with lemon juice, tamari, almond butter, water and coconut milk in a blender until smooth. Now put chicken and broccoli in a frying pan and spread the mixture over it. Cover the pan and cook it for 15 minutes. Your dish is ready. Garnish it with nuts and cranberries to serve.

*Detailed nutritional breakup of the recipe:

Nutritional Value For Each Recipe: Chicken with Coconut & Almond: Serving Size: 6.					
/TOTAL CALORIES	128.4	/Vitamin-A	86.4 RE	Potassium	655.5 mg

/TOTAL FAT	11.3g	/Vitamin-C	52.9 mg	Zinc	2.1mg
/SATURATED FAT	1.7g	/Thiamin (B-1)	0.1mg	Magnesium	124.5 mg
/CARBO-HYDRATE	6.2g	/Riboflavin (B-2)	0.3mg	Phosphorus	362.8 mg
/FIBER	2.6g	/Vitamin B-12	0.3µg	Iron	3.2mg
/CHOLESTEROL	0.0mg	/Vitamin B-6	0.7mg	Calcium	115.7 mg
/PROTEIN	2.9g	/Niacin	11.8 mg	Vitamin-E	0.3mg
/SODIUM	293mg	/Folate	64.8µg	Vitamin-D	0µg

As you can see in the nutritional chart, this dish is full of nutritional support, so it is better to add this dish to your regular meal chart.

Super food – Quinoa:

Dr. Erika Siegel has termed this food item as a "prescription of nutrients for PA patients and everyone else." As we know, quinoa is one of the most popular super foods. Quinoa is full of minerals, fibre, and protein. Quinoa is also gluten-free, which makes it ideal for weight control and nutritional balance. Let me point out some health benefits of Quinoa at this point, to emphasise patients of Psoriatic arthritis to use it as a regular ingredient in their meals.

Quinoa Benefits for Psoriatic Arthritis:

(1) – It has low calories i.e. about 222 only in 1 cup of quinoa grains, with very low percentage of fats (4g) and carbs (39g). Patients suffering with Psoriatic arthritis, obesity and stomach-burn can use it on a regular basis.

(2) – It has rich nutritious value with Manganese (58% of the Recommended Dietary Allowance (RDA), Iron (15% of the RDA), Magnesium (30% of the RDA), Folate (19% of the RDA), Copper (18% of the RDA), Potassium (9% of the RDA), Iron

(15% of the RDA), Vitamins B1, B2 and B6 (over 10% of RDA) and Vitamin-E, Vitamin-B3 and Calcium in small amounts.

(3) – Quercetin and Kaempferol: Quinoa is rich in flavonoids that act as anti-inflammatory and antioxidants. The two most effective and known types of flavonoids present in quinoa are Quercetin and Kaempferol. Several animal studies have shown that these two flavonoids can have positive effects as anti-depressants, anti-viral and anti-inflammatory agents.

(4) – Just like all other grains, quinoa is also rich in fibre. In fact, the fibre content is greater than most of the other grains with 17-27 grams fibre per cup.

(5) – Essential Amino Acids & Low Glycaemic index: There are certain types of essential amino acids like Lysine that the human body cannot produce on its own. So, we need to consume these amino acids via an external food source. Quinoa is a proven, rich source of essential amino acids. Quinoa is also a better option for patients having elevated blood sugar levels (diabetes) and heart diseases due to its low glycaemic index.

(6) – Healthy Metabolic Rate: A couple of studies have shown that quinoa can be a healthy choice in order to reduce fructose intake and improve metabolic rate.

You can find and try several quinoa-based recipes on the web. Let me remind you again that quinoa is good for your health if you are a PA patient or not.

2. Easy to Cook Chicken:

There are some dishes in this book you cannot stop yourself from eating. And "easy to cook chicken" is certainly one among many. It is easy to cook and impressive indeed. Ideal for serving six or more.

Ingredients: - Yams (1½ pounds, sliced), - rice wine vinegar (1 cup), - miso paste (1½ tablespoons), - organic chicken broth (1½ cups), - dried thyme (1 teaspoon), - garlic powder (1 tablespoon), - onion (1 large, sliced), - carrots (5 large, quartered) – you can replace with 25 baby carrots as well, - cayenne pepper (according to your taste), - dried parsley (2 tablespoons), - organic chicken breasts (6 to 8 boneless, skinless pieces that will be around 3 pounds in total), and - olive oil (3 tablespoons).

How to prepare: First of all, preheat your oven at 475°F. Using a bowl, mix miso paste, chicken broth, rice wine, vinegar, thyme, and garlic powder together. Once the vegetables are sliced, place them on a baking dish. The size of the baking dish should be around 13 x 9-inches. Marinate the chicken with the mixture after placing it onto the dish with sliced vegetables. Now sprinkle cayenne pepper, parsley and olive oil over. Place the dish in the oven and bake it for about 1 hour until brown. Remember to turn the chicken over after 30 minutes so that it is evenly baked from both sides. Your dish is ready to serve with brown rice or green salad.

*Detailed nutritional breakup of the recipe:

Nutritional Value For Each Recipe:					
Easy to Cook Chicken: Serving Size: 6					
/TOTAL CALORIES	510.5	/Vitamin-A	2894.1 RE	Potassium	1837.4 mg
/TOTAL FAT	10.3 g	/Vitamin-C	24.6 mg	Zinc	2.5mg
/SATURATED FAT	1.8g	/Thiamin (B-1)	0.3 mg	Magnesium	89.5 mg
/CARBO-HYDRATE	46.6g	/Riboflavin (B-2)	0.3 Mg	Phosphorus	533.8 mg
/FIBER	8.4g	/Vitamin B-12	1.5 µg	Iron	3.3mg
/CHOLESTEROL	131.4 mg	/Vitamin B-6	0.6 mg	Calcium	97.8 mg
/PROTEIN	56.3g	/Niacin	22.0 Mg	Vitamin-E	0.0mg
/SODIUM	475.7 mg	/Folate	51.0 µg	Vitamin-D	0.0µg

3. Nut & Lentil Loaf:

This is the best option for vegetarians. People wanting to consume more vegetables can take this loaf with salad or roasted vegetables. Very anti-inflammatory in nature, thus ideal for the Psoriatic arthritis diet.

Ingredients: - Cooked brown rice (2 cups), - garlic (8 cloves, cut in half), - olive oil (1 tablespoon of extra-virgin), - walnuts (2 cups, ground), - dried lentils (8 ounces), - onion (1 large, chopped), - teriyaki sauce (2 tablespoons), - organic eggs (two), - mashed banana (half), - oregano (2 teaspoons), - fresh parsley (3 tablespoons, chopped), - sea salt (according to your taste), - black pepper (according to your taste).

How to cook: all lentils should be soaked 3 hours prior to cooking. Fry chopped onions until brown in a small pan with extra virgin olive oil. Mix all ingredients in a loaf pan and bake it for 1 hour or until cooked. Serving size is normally four people.

*Detailed nutritional breakup of the recipe:

Nutritional Value For Each Recipe:					
Nut & Lentil Loaf: Serving Size: 6					
/TOTAL CALORIES	541.2	/Vitamin-A	48.9 RE	Potassium	607.5 mg
/TOTAL FAT	31.1 g	/Vitamin-C	97.4 mg	Zinc	3.6mg
/SATURATED FAT	3.5g	/Thiamin (B-1)	0.5 mg	Magnesium	141.5 mg
/CARBO-HYDRATE	50.1g	/Riboflavin (B-2)	0.3 mg	Phosphorus	402.2 mg
/FIBER	16.3g	/Vitamin B-12	0.2 µg	Iron	4.7mg
/CHOLESTEROL	70.5 mg	/Vitamin B-6	0.6 mg	Calcium	97.4 mg
/PROTEIN	20.6g	/Niacin	2.4 Mg	Vitamin-E	0.0mg
/SODIUM	262 mg	/Folate	151.2 µg	Vitamin-D	0.2µg

4. Easy Stir Fry:

Some people find cooking very difficult while others think of it as an art that only few people can master. I love eating but am very amateur at cooking. This recipe is special for those who are not good at cooking. It is a very simple and quick dish to prepare within minutes. One can also add or try different vegetables to bring variety and taste. Stir-fry dishes can taste similar very quickly so it is important to try multiple options. Luckily, this dish allows you complete creativity and choice of taste.

Ingredients: - Onion (1 medium, minced), - olive oil (2 tablespoons), - zucchini (1 cup, sliced), - garlic cloves (take two, minced), - carrots (3 large, sliced evenly), - crimini mushrooms (use eight, sliced), - green pepper (one large, chopped), - sea salt (according to your taste), - pepper (according to your taste), - wheat-free tamari (2 tablespoons), and - other seasonings to taste.

Instructions: Fry chopped onions and garlic in a pan until soft. Put seasonings and vegetables to the pan and stir often. Cook until the vegetables get crispy. The dish is ready to serve and eat. This is how simple the dish is to make.

*Detailed nutritional breakup of the recipe:

Nutritional Value For Each Recipe:					
Easy Stir Fry: Serving Size: 4					
/TOTAL CALORIES	112.8	/Vitamin-A	1315.4 RE	Potassium	337.2 mg
/TOTAL FAT	7.0 g	/Vitamin-C	33.6 mg	Zinc	0.3mg
/SATURATED FAT	1.0g	/Thiamin (B-1)	0.1 mg	Magnesium	20 mg
/CARBO-HYDRATE	11g	/Riboflavin (B-2)	0.1 mg	Phosphorus	54.1 mg
/FIBER	2.9g	/Vitamin B-12	0.0 µg	Iron	0.8mg
/CHOLESTEROL	0.0 mg	/Vitamin B-6	0.3 mg	Calcium	32.9 mg
/PROTEIN	2.9g	/Niacin	1.1	Vitamin-E	0.0mg

			mg		
/SODIUM	544.7 mg	/Folate	27.1 µg	Vitamin-D	0.0µg

(7) Salads

I consider this as one of the most usable and beneficial parts of the diet section. Salads are rich in nutrition, but above all, they are always easy and quick to make. All the salads in this book are healthy, nutritious and full of taste.

1. Avocado-Bean Salad:

The best thing you will find in this book is information about the most beneficial food items. In addition, the information is mostly research-based and clinically proven. *Avocado* is another top healthy food item that everyone should eat on a regular basis due to its outstanding fitness value. The use of the avocado tree has been so popular that its leaves, stem, fruit and seeds are used to make various medicines. The fruit is famous for stimulating menstrual flow, lower cholesterol levels, treating osteoarthritis and enhancing sexual desire. Avocado also has a beneficial role to play for Psoriasis and Psoriatic arthritis patients. *Avocado oil* and vitamin-B12 are used in combination to treat Psoriasis (a skin condition, potentially leading to Psoriatic arthritis). Avocado has additional uses as well. For example: seeds, leaves, bark and fruit palp can be used to speed up wound healing, treat toothache and diarrhoea, and accelerate hair growth.

Ingredients: - Cooked pinto beans (3 cups, you can use 3 different kinds of beans at the same time to add more nutritional content to your salad like black, kidney, green, garbanzo or others), - avocados (2 large ripe, peeled and cut into small cubes), - lettuce leaves (six large, for serving), - red pepper (½ cup, chopped), - green pepper (½ cup, chopped).

Ingredients for Dressing: - Rice vinegar (2/3cup), - olive oil (2/3cup), - fresh parsley (2 teaspoons, chopped), - raw honey (3 tablespoons), - fresh coriander leaves (2 teaspoons chopped, cilantro), - black pepper (½ teaspoon or according to taste).

Instructions to prepare: start by mixing the beans, avocado and peppers in a bowl. Now mix the dressing items in a separate bowl. Remember to reserve some parsley for later use as dressing.. In order to serve, put salad on top of lettuce leaves. The salad is ready to eat. Sprinkle parsley before serving.

*Detailed nutritional breakup of the recipe:

Nutritional Value For Each Recipe:					
Avocado-Bean Salad: Serving Size: 4					
/TOTAL CALORIES	476.9	/Vitamin-A	122.7 RE	Potassium	723.4 mg
/TOTAL FAT	34.1 g	/Vitamin-C	40.9 mg	Zinc	1.3mg
/SATURATED FAT	4.7g	/Thiamin (B-1)	0.2 mg	Magnesium	63.7 mg
/CARBO-HYDRATE	37.5g	/Riboflavin (B-2)	0.2 mg	Phosphorus	164.3 mg
/FIBER	12.1g	/Vitamin B-12	0.0 µg	Iron	2.7mg
/CHOLESTEROL	0.0 mg	/Vitamin B-6	0.4 mg	Calcium	56.4 mg
/PROTEIN	9.2g	/Niacin	2.7 mg	Vitamin-E	3.8mg
/SODIUM	8.3 mg	/Folate	189.9 µg	Vitamin-D	0.0µg

2. Beet-Bean Salad:

Let's talk about the health benefits of beet before getting to the recipe. Several medicines are produced using beet plant and its roots. Its most impressive role is evident in obese individuals. The reason behind is that it can help lower blood pressure, lower the level of triglycerides, enhance athletic performance and treat some certain types of liver dysfunction.

Recipe: - Beets (3 to 4 large size, make sure beets are well steamed until tender and peeled), - hazelnuts (¼ cup), - green beans (1½ cups, cut into small cubes and make sure that beans are also well steamed until tender), - leek (one, sliced – try to use the white part), - pear (one, cut into thin slices), - white beans (one cup, cooked).

Ingredients for Dressing: - Olive oil (¼ cup extra virgin), - garlic (2 cloves, minced), - fresh dill (2 tablespoons) or dry dill (1 teaspoon), - mustard (2 teaspoons – keeping in mind that there are no additives or added sugar in it), - balsamic vinegar (2 teaspoons).

Instructions: Start by cooking the beets. Once cooked, cut the beets in small pieces. Now, mix leek slices, green beans, white beans and pear slices in a large bowl. Coming to the dressing part, mix all dressing ingredients that include garlic, mustard, fresh oil, balsamic vinegar and extra-virgin olive oil and your dressing is ready. Pour the dressing over the salad and whip. Once the mixture is marinated in the dressing, put it in the refrigerator for about 1 hour. Sprinkle hazelnuts before serving.

*Detailed nutritional breakup of the recipe:

Nutritional Value For Each Recipe: Beet-Bean Salad: Serving Size: 6					
/TOTAL CALORIES	215.5	/Vitamin-A	22.1 RE	Potassium	457.1 mg
/TOTAL FAT	13.2g	/Vitamin-C	9.2mg	Zinc	0.8mg
/SATURATED FAT	1.6g	/Thiamin (B-1)	0.1mg	Magnesium	51mg
/CARBO-HYDRATE	21.4g	/Riboflavin (B-2)	0mg	Phosphorus	87.1 mg
/FIBER	5.3g	/Vitamin B-12	0µg	Iron	2.5mg
/CHOLESTEROL	0.0mg	/Vitamin B-6	0.2mg	Calcium	65.5 mg

/PROTEIN	5.4g	/Niacin	1.0mg	Vitamin-E	1.3mg
/SODIUM	58mg	/Folate	93.4µg	Vitamin-D	0µg

3. Tasty & Colourful Shredded Cabbage:

Some recipes are better than others and some are exceptional. Recipes having cabbage in the ingredient list are ideal for people looking to lose weight. Cabbage has multiple health benefits and burning fat is just one. Cabbage is also good for osteoarthritis (all types of weak bones), asthma, morning sickness, stomach pain and different types of cancer including stomach cancer, lung cancer, colon cancer and breast cancer. However, diabetes patients should be conscious in consuming cabbage in large quantities.

Ingredients: - Fresh cilantro (2 tablespoons), - flaxseed oil or olive oil (3 tablespoons), - red wine vinegar (2 tablespoons), - lemon juice (1 tablespoon), - honey (1 tablespoon), - white cabbage (2 cups – shredded), - red cabbage (2 cups – shredded), - carrots (three – shredded), - apple (one – shredded), - boiling water (4 cups), - raisins (¼ cup - optional; exclude if you are diabetic), - onion (half - chopped), - horseradish (1 teaspoon - from a jar), - garlic powder 9¼ teaspoon), - onion powder (¼ teaspoon), - sea salt (according to your taste) or tamari (optional)

How to Cook: Put cabbage in a large bowl. Add raisins to it. Now add boiling water and cover for 5 minutes. It's time to drain the water and mix all ingredients with the cabbage. Allow it to refrigerate for about two hours. Your salad is ready to serve. Try multiple substitutions in this salad that will allow for different taste and nutritional benefits. For example: add more apple or honey to make the salad sweeter. You can also replace raisins with apples.

*Detailed nutritional breakup of the recipe:

Nutritional Value For Each Recipe: Tasty & Colourful Shredded Cabbage: Serving Size: 6

74

/TOTAL CALORIES	117.0	/Vitamin-A	1141.7 RE	Potassium	270.4 mg
/TOTAL FAT	7.3g	/Vitamin-C	27.3 mg	Zinc	0.2mg
/SATURATED FAT	1.0g	/Thiamin (B-1)	0.1mg	Magnesium	14.9 mg
/CARBO-HYDRATE	13.4g	/Riboflavin (B-2)	0mg	Phosphorus	37.0 mg
/FIBER	2.6g	/Vitamin B-12	0µg	Iron	0.6mg
/CHOLES-TEROL	0.0mg	/Vitamin B-6	0.1mg	Calcium	37.6 mg
/PROTEIN	1.2g	/Niacin	0.9mg	Vitamin-E	1.1mg
/SODIUM	24.5mg	/Folate	22.3µg	Vitamin-D	0µg

4. Lettuce-Chicken Salad:

This is a very famous Indian recipe. It is full of flavours, colours and nutrition. This salad can be eaten as a complete meal to provide the body with all food requirements. You can also enjoy and serve it to your guests with several main dishes. Everyone will certainly love this one.

Ingredients: - Mayonnaise (½ cup organic - one with natural ingredients), - diced celery (½ cup), - chicken breast (1¼ pounds, (remember to take organic chicken from farmers' stores) baked and cubed, - lettuce leaves (6 large)- Fuji apple (½ medium), - raisins (¼–½ cup), - salt (½ teaspoon or according to taste), - black pepper (according to taste), - onion (¼ cup - diced),- curry powder (2½ teaspoons), and - turmeric (½ teaspoon).

Instructions: Put all the ingredients in a large mixing bowl and whip. Once mixed together, refrigerate the salad for 30 minutes to 1 hour. Now serve chilled on lettuce leaves.

*Detailed nutritional breakup of the recipe:

Nutritional Value For Each Recipe: Lettuce-Chicken Salad: Serving Size: 4					
/TOTAL	412.2	/Vitamin-	29.6	Potassium	623.3

CALORIES		A	RE		mg
/TOTAL FAT	24.9 g	/Vitamin-C	5.4 mg	Zinc	1.3mg
/SATURATED FAT	2.8g	/Thiamin (B-1)	0.1 mg	Magnesium	52.4 mg
/CARBO-HYDRATE	13g	/Riboflavin (B-2)	0.2 mg	Phosphorus	32.6 mg
/FIBER	1.5g	/Vitamin B-12	0.6 µg	Iron	1.6mg
/CHOLESTEROL	98.5 mg	/Vitamin B-6	0.8 mg	Calcium	34.3 mg
/PROTEIN	33.5g	/Niacin	16.1 mg	Vitamin-E	1.4mg
/SODIUM	530.5 mg	/Folate	32.6 µg	Vitamin-D	0.1µg

5. Bean-Garlic Salad:

Spices and herbs can play a vital role in our health and inflammation control. Most of the common herbs and spices we use in daily life (especially Mediterranean & Asian region) are all either antiseptic or antibiotics naturally. These virile characteristics allow us to have taste along with several health benefits.

The health benefits of Garlic:

Garlic is a very commonly used herb and a flavouring agent in most Asian dishes. Recently, garlic has become a potent ingredient in several medicines and supplements. The Chinese have a very long history of using herbs in their traditional medicine and garlic is no exception. Garlic is well reputed to have multiple health benefits for us. Garlic can be effective for the treatment and prevention of the following: - Stomach inflammation (gastritis), - Hardening of the arteries (atherosclerosis), - Rectal cancer, - Stomach cancer, - High blood pressure, - Jock itch, - Athlete's foot, - Lumpy breast tissue (fibrocystic breast disease), - Hepatitis, - Ringworm, - Corns, - Tick bites, - Chest pain, - Hair loss, - Benign prostatic hyperplasia

76

(BPH), - Clogged arteries (coronary heart disease), - Cancer in the esophagus, - Low athletic performance, - Common cold, - Shortness of breath, - Tightening & hardening of the skin (scleroderma), - Warts, - Liver disease (hepatopulmonary syndrome), - Lead poisoning, - Cancer of bone marrow cells (like multiple myeloma), - Thrush (oral candidiasis), - Prostate cancer.

The following recipe is full of healthy ingredients like garlic, olive oil, apple cider vinegar and thyme. Try to add this recipe to your weekly menu. It is also helpful for people looking to shred some unwanted fat.

Ingredients: - Olive oil (2 tablespoons), - apple cider vinegar (2 teaspoons), - garlic clove (one, minced), - green beans (1 pound, blanched & cooled), - thyme (½ teaspoon), - shallot (1 small, minced), - sea salt, and - pepper.

How to cook: Cook beans until bright green and then allow it to cool. Add all remaining ingredients with green beans and mix well. Serve chilled and enjoy!

*Detailed nutritional breakup of the recipe:

Nutritional Value For Each Recipe:					
Bean-Garlic Salad: Serving Size: 4					
/TOTAL CALORIES	101.1	/Vitamin-A	81.7 RE	Potassium	223.9 mg
/TOTAL FAT	7.2 g	/Vitamin-C	14.3 mg	Zinc	0.3mg
/SATURATED FAT	1.0g	/Thiamin (B-1)	0.1 mg	Magnesium	28.3 mg
/CARBO-HYDRATE	8.8g	/Riboflavin (B-2)	0.1 mg	Phosphorus	41.2 mg
/FIBER	3.9g	/Vitamin B-12	0.0 µg	Iron	1.5mg
/CHOLESTEROL	0.0 mg	/Vitamin B-6	0.1 mg	Calcium	46.1 mg
/PROTEIN	2.2g	/Niacin	1.1 mg	Vitamin-E	0.8mg
/SODIUM	7.3 mg	/Folate	28.0 µg	Vitamin-D	0.0µg

6. Tuna-Avocado Salad:

Some diet foods are so nutritious and healthy that they can be seen in nearly all healthy diets. Avocado and Tuna are both among such healthy foods. We have already mentioned several health benefits of avocado and its potential benefits for psoriatic arthritis as well. Let's have a quick overview about the usefulness of tuna.

Tuna: If you want to add a food in your recipe list that is full of vitamins, minerals and healthy nutrients then you should go for tuna fish. You will find multiple positives about, and rarely any negative points, for tuna fish.

(1) – It is loaded with proteins but contains very few saturated fats. Proteins in tuna fish are also good for nails, hair and skin.

(2) – If taken in moderation, it can lower the risk of a stroke to 27 to 30 per cent in general population.

(3) – Tuna fish is also an excellent source of omega 3 fatty acids. Omega 3 fatty acids are good for keeping blood pressure in control, preventing heart-related disorders.

(4) – Triglyceride levels set the parameters for fat quantity in the bloodstream. High triglyceride levels are also associated with bad cholesterol (low-density lipoprotein-LDL). Consuming tuna twice a week can help you lower your bad cholesterol level.

(5) – Heart rate variability (HRV) or simply known as heartbeat is crucial to maintain a healthy heart and smooth blood pressure. There are several aspects involved. Nevertheless, eating tuna is a proven remedy for a steady heartbeat.

(6) – Being overweight/obese can be most benefited by eating tuna. Tuna will allow the regulation of a metabolic hormone named leptin through omega-3 fatty acids. Leptin can play a vital role in maintaining healthy weight and food intake. Therefore, tuna and other seafood that is rich in omega-3 fatty acids can be

helpful for weight loss and long term targeted weight maintenance.

(7) – There are a few basic systems in our body that run and control all crucial functions. Our immune system is one of these basic but very fundamental systems. It is responsible for preventing and curing all kinds of diseases and internal and external threats. Tuna is rich in selenium, which is a proven antioxidant. Antioxidants like selenium are significant to eliminate toxins from our body and to make our immune system strong. High immunity means long lasting health.

(8) – Essential nutrients are important for normal growth, especially in children and adolescents. Tuna is loaded with micronutrients like vitamin-B. Vitamin-B can induce steady blood pressure, improved immune system, healthy skin and stabilised metabolism.

(9) – Tuna can be helpful in the prevention and treatment of some fatal chronic diseases like cancer. Multiple research studies have shown that tuna can play a part in reducing the risk of kidney cancer. Tuna has a low amount of calories and saturated fats, so it can be a better replacement for dairy products.

(10) – There are some health concerns associated with the increased intake of tuna. For example, tuna contains a high content of sodium and mercury. Both can result in high blood pressure and kidney problems. Fortunately, eating tuna in moderation can easily eliminate any potential risks.

Ingredients (Tuna-Avocado Salad):

- Medium avocado (1 ripe),

- Light tuna (12 ounce – probably two cans of 6 ounce each),

- Pepper (¼–½ teaspoon or according to your taste)

- Sea salt (½ teaspoon - optional).

How to prepare: First start by mashing avocado. Once you are done then add tuna and pepper. Whip together and serve it over lettuce leaves, or with non-wheat bread, on rice crackers or green salad.

*Detailed nutritional breakup of the recipe:

Nutritional Value For Each Recipe: Tuna-Avocado Salad: Serving Size: 4				
/TOTAL CALORIES	222.7	/Vitamin-A	53.9 RE	Potassium	545.8 mg
/TOTAL FAT	9.2 g	/Vitamin-C	5.7 mg	Zinc	1.2mg
/SATURATED FAT	1.5g	/Thiamin (B-1)	0.1 mg	Magnesium	47.4 mg
/CARBO-HYDRATE	4.9g	/Riboflavin (B-2)	0.2 mg	Phosphorus	214.6 mg
/FIBER	3.8g	/Vitamin B-12	3.4 µg	Iron	2.1mg
/CHOLESTEROL	34.0 mg	/Vitamin B-6	0.5 mg	Calcium	20 mg
/PROTEIN	30.1g	/Niacin	16.0 mg	Vitamin-E	0.8mg
/SODIUM	387.3 mg	/Folate	37.4 µg	Vitamin-D	0.0µg

7. Continental Carrot Salad:

First of all, a specific diet recipe for psoriatic arthritis or any other types of inflammatory diseases should have healthy and easily available ingredients. A continuous voice about the necessity of vegetables and fruits for psoriatic arthritis has been spread over the years. However, most of the times it is very hard to find a healthy vegetable-based recipe that is both full of taste and nutrition. For all above reasons, continental carrot salad must be rated high due to its great taste and health advantages.

Health Uses & Benefits of Carrot: This is a plant that has several health uses. Its seeds are a good source of oil used in making certain medicine. There is also a wild type of carrot, which is not edible. General health uses of carrots include: Bladder problems, Cancer, Water retention, Gout, Diarrhoea, Indigestion, Gas,

Worm infestations, Use as an aphrodisiac, Starting menstruation (periods), Pain in the uterus, Heart disease, Use as a nerve tonic, Kidney stones and other kidney problems.

Anti-Aging effects: It can act as a perfect anti-aging agent due to the presence of beta-carotene (a potent antioxidant). Beta-carotene can certainly limit oxidative-stress and reduce cell damage.

Prevention of Chronic Disorders: Scientists have discovered falcarinol and falcarindiol in carrots that can reduce the risk of colon cancer, lung cancer and breast cancer.

Optimal Vision: Beta-carotene (active form of vitamin-A) is good for the eyes. It acts on the retina (as rhodopsin, a purple pigment) to improve vision.

Beautiful Glowing Skin: The mixture of grated carrot and honey makes a wonderful anti-wrinkle mask for the face, hands and feet.

Body Cleansing & Detoxification: carrots are a good source of fibre. Carrot fibre is good for colon cleansing and helps in waste movement. Vitamin rich carrots can also improve liver function by reducing bile and fat in the liver.

Preventing Stroke & Heart-related Disorders: A research study conducted by Harvard University suggested that people eating six carrots per week are less likely to have stroke. Lutein, alpha-carotene and beta-carotene are all associated with the reduced risk of heart-related disorders.

Ingredients (Continental Carrot Salad): - Extra virgin olive oil (2 tablespoons), - carrots (1 pound - cut into 3 inch-long and thin sticks), - red wine vinegar (2 tablespoons), - dried basil (1 teaspoon), - garlic cloves (3 - minced fine), - sea salt and pepper (according to taste).

Instructions:

1. First, put all the carrot into a steamer and steam the sticks until crisp-tender.

2. Secondly, mix together all remaining ingredients in a mixing bowl.

3. Now, add the above mixture and carrots in a sealable container. Seal it and allow it to cool in a refrigerator for some time (up to 1 hour or overnight).

4. Remember to turn around the position of the container periodically.

5. The salad is ready, serve chilled.

*Detailed nutritional breakup of the recipe:

Nutritional Value For Each Recipe:					
Continental Carrot Salad: Serving Size: 4					
/TOTAL CALORIES	116.4	/Vitamin-A	2885 RE	Potassium	388.7 mg
/TOTAL FAT	7.3 g	/Vitamin-C	8.9 mg	Zinc	0.3mg
/SATURATED FAT	1.0g	/Thiamin (B-1)	0.1 mg	Magnesium	19.1 mg
/CARBO-HYDRATE	12.5g	/Riboflavin (B-2)	0.1 mg	Phosphorus	55.2 mg
/FIBER	3.0g	/Vitamin B-12	0.0 µg	Iron	0.8mg
/CHOLESTEROL	0.0 mg	/Vitamin B-6	0.2 mg	Calcium	43.2 mg
/PROTEIN	1.4g	/Niacin	1.4 mg	Vitamin-E	1.4mg
/SODIUM	40.8 mg	/Folate	13.8 µg	Vitamin-D	0.0µg

8. Carrot-Beet Salad:

Ingredients: - Raw beets (three, peeled and grated), - carrots (½ pound, grated), - apple cider vinegar (4 tablespoons), - extra virgin olive oil (3 tablespoons), - mustard (2 tablespoons - no additives/sugar), - pepper (¼ teaspoon), and - sea salt (¼ teaspoon).

How to cook: Take grated beets and grated carrots in a mixing bowl. Put all dressing ingredients in the bowl and mix well. You can put it in the refrigerator in order to serve chilled.

*Detailed nutritional breakup of the recipe:

Nutritional Value For Each Recipe: Carrot-Beet Salad: Serving Size: 4					
/TOTAL CALORIES	156.1	/Vitamin-A	1443.3 RE	Potassium	410.2 mg
/TOTAL FAT	11.4 g	/Vitamin-C	7.0 mg	Zinc	0.4mg
/SATURATED FAT	1.6g	/Thiamin (B-1)	0.1 mg	Magnesium	27.7 mg
/CARBO-HYDRATE	13.0g	/Riboflavin (B-2)	0.1 mg	Phosphorus	63.0 mg
/FIBER	2.7g	/Vitamin B-12	0.0 µg	Iron	1.2mg
/CHOLESTEROL	0.0 Mg	/Vitamin B-6	0.1 mg	Calcium	39.2 mg
/PROTEIN	2.1g	/Niacin	1.2 mg	Vitamin-E	2.1mg
/SODIUM	329.8 mg	/Folate	73.3 µg	Vitamin-D	0.0µg

9. Spinach-Honey-Lemon Salad:

Ingredients: - Fresh spinach (4 cups), - lemon juice (about 3–4 lemons), - honey (½ cup), - grated lemon zest (2 teaspoons), - sea salt (1 teaspoon), and - cayenne pepper (according to your taste).

Instructions: Add all the ingredients along with fresh spinach in a mixing bowl and whip well. Toss gently and your salad is ready to serve.

*Detailed nutritional breakup of the recipe:

Nutritional Value For Each Recipe: Spinach-Honey-Lemon Salad: Serving Size: 6					
/TOTAL	145.2	/Vitamin-A	202.5	Potassium	241.4

CALORIES			RE		mg
/TOTAL FAT	0.1g	/Vitamin-C	28.6 mg	Zinc	0.3mg
/SATURATED FAT	0g	/Thiamin (B-1)	0.0mg	Magnesium	27.1 mg
/CARBO-HYDRATE	39.4g	/Riboflavin (B-2)	0.1mg	Phosphorus	18.9 mg
/FIBER	1.0g	/Vitamin B-12	0µg	Iron	1.0mg
/CHOLESTEROL	0.0mg	/Vitamin B-6	0.1mg	Calcium	36.8 mg
/PROTEIN	1.1g	/Niacin	0.3mg	Vitamin-E	0mg
/SODIUM	607.2 mg	/Folate	64.4µg	Vitamin-D	0µg

Uses of Spinach for Psoriatic Patients:

Just like Popeye, every kid and adult in the modern age can benefit from the wonders of spinach.

1. *Trace minerals & Micronutrients*: Spinach is the number 1 food to have most nutrients per calorie. It is rich in micronutrients like vitamin-A, vitamin-K, vitamin-D3 and several trace elements.

2. *Omega 3 Fatty Acids*: Spinach contains omega-3 fatty acids that are essential to several major organs in our body. Omega-3 fatty acids can be influential in the following medical conditions: blood fat (triglycerides), rheumatoid arthritis, depression and anxiety, neurological development in new-born babies, asthma, ADHD, memory loss, dementia and Alzheimer's disease.

3. *Alkalises the Human Body*: High acid diets can lead to obesity, energy drainage and several other medical complications. Spinach provides the necessary alkaline to neutralise the negative aspects of acidic diets.

4. *Powerful Bones & Eyes*: macular degeneration and cataracts are two common eye-related complications that can be prevented and cured with the regular intake of spinach. Selenium, calcium and vitamin-K in spinach can provide optimal bone strength for long lasting health.

(8) Savoury Soups

1. Delicious Mushroom Soup:

Ingredients: - Celery stalks (4 – chopped), - extra virgin olive oil 93 tablespoons), - onions (2 medium, chopped), - garlic (six cloves, minced), - dried rosemary (1 tablespoon), - dried sage (1 tablespoon), - shiitake mushrooms (2 cups – sliced), - crimini mushrooms (2 cups – sliced), - organic chicken broth (7 cups), - yellow miso paste (3 tablespoons), - bay leaves (three), - dried thyme (1 tablespoon), - large carrots (four – chopped), - black pepper (as per taste), and - sea salt (as per taste).

Cooking instructions: Put onions, garlic, celery, rosemary, thyme and sage in a big pan and cook slightly over a medium heat until celery and onions are semi-transparent. Now, add mushrooms and carrots and cook for another 3 minutes. After cooking for another 1 minute, add bay leaves and miso paste. Now simmer the ingredients for about 25 to 30 minutes. At the end, add sea salt and pepper according to your taste.

*Detailed nutritional breakup of the recipe:

Nutritional Value For Each Recipe:					
Delicious Mushroom Soup: Serving Size: 4					
/TOTAL CALORIES	191.6	/Vitamin-A	1667.4 RE	Potassium	703.7 mg
/TOTAL FAT	8.4 g	/Vitamin-C	11.5 mg	Zinc	1.1mg
/SATURATED FAT	1.1g	/Thiamin (B-1)	0.1 mg	Magnesium	30.4 mg
/CARBO-HYDRATE	27.7g	/Riboflavin (B-2)	0.2 mg	Phosphorus	360.2 mg

/FIBER	5.7g	/Vitamin B-12	0.0 µg	Iron	2.7mg
/CHOLESTEROL	0.0 Mg	/Vitamin B-6	0.3 mg	Calcium	99.7 mg
/PROTEIN	5.0g	/Niacin	1.9 mg	Vitamin-E	1.2mg
/SODIUM	714.3 mg	/Folate	33.6 µg	Vitamin-D	0.0µg

2. Awesome Winter Soup:

Ingredients: - Olive oil (2 tablespoons), - onion (half, chopped), - turmeric root (¼ cup chopped) or turmeric powder (½teaspoon), - butternut squash (½ medium - peeled & cubed), - carrots (4 medium, sliced thinly), - burdock root (1/3cup sliced), - grated fresh ginger (4 tablespoons), - garlic (8 cloves, chopped), - vegetable stock (8 cups), - fresh parsley (2 tablespoons, chopped), - salt (to taste), - lemon slices (three only), - whole leaves of kale (4, chopped), - miso paste (¼ cup), - cayenne pepper (1 teaspoon), - curry powder (1 teaspoon), and - green onions (¼ cup - sliced, for garnish).

Cooking details: Use a large soup pot to sauté turmeric root, carrots, burdock and squash in extra virgin olive oil. Sauté these ingredients for 8 to 10 minutes at medium-high heat until soft. Later, add ginger, garlic and onions and cook for another 5 minutes. It's time to add kale, parsley, lemon slices, cayenne, curry, salt and vegetable stock and cook for a further 40 minutes at medium-low heat. The soup is ready. Now add miso paste and stir well. Sprinkle garnish (green onions) before serving.

*Detailed nutritional breakup of the recipe:

Nutritional Value For Each Recipe:					
Awesome Winter Soup: Serving Size: 4					
/TOTAL CALORIES	262.5	/Vitamin-A	3124.4 RE	Potassium	1221.2 mg
/TOTAL FAT	9.7	/Vitamin-	41.8	Zinc	1.0mg

	g	C	mg		
/SATURATED FAT	1.3g	/Thiamin (B-1)	0.2 mg	Magnesium	60.6 mg
/CARBO-HYDRATE	39.5g	/Riboflavin (B-2)	0.1 mg	Phosphorus	769.1 mg
/FIBER	7.8g	/Vitamin B-12	0.0 µg	Iron	2.9mg
/CHOLESTEROL	0.0 Mg	/Vitamin B-6	0.4 mg	Calcium	145.4 mg
/PROTEIN	6.9g	/Niacin	2.4 mg	Vitamin-E	1.3mg
/SODIUM	1600.6 mg	/Folate	43.8 µg	Vitamin-D	0.0µg

3. *Tongue-Teaser Lemon-Coconut Soup*:

Ingredients: - Extra virgin olive oil (2 teaspoons), - red onion (half - cut into very thin rings), - chicken breasts (about 1½ pounds or two pieces - cubed), - honey (1 tablespoon + 1 teaspoon), - light coconut milk (one: 13.5-ounce can), - lemongrass (3 stalks, cut into large chunks (for flavour purposes only and not to be eaten), - hot chilli (one, minced & seeded), - dried cayenne pepper (2 generous dashes-optional), - small mushrooms (10, sliced thinly), - filtered water (1 cup), - juice of lemon (½ medium size lemon), - fish sauce (2 teaspoons), and - galangal root (optional).

Cooking instructions: Sauté the red onion in a saucepan along with chicken until onions are translucent. Keeping the coconut milk aside, add all the remaining ingredients and cook for 15 minutes. After that, add coconut milk and simmer for another 15 minutes. Do not boil coconut milk or it will separate. Cook until vegetables and chicken done. Tasty and nutritious *Tongue-Teaser Lemon-Coconut Soup* is ready to serve and eat.

*Detailed nutritional breakup of the recipe:

Nutritional Value For Each Recipe:

Tongue-Teaser Lemon-Coconut Soup: Serving Size: 4					
/TOTAL CALORIES	323.0	/Vitamin-A	132.6 RE	Potassium	745.0 mg
/TOTAL FAT	11.1 g	/Vitamin-C	37.6 mg	Zinc	1.5mg
/SATURATED FAT	4.6g	/Thiamin (B-1)	0.2 mg	Magnesium	58.8 mg
/CARBO-HYDRATE	14.6g	/Riboflavin (B-2)	0.4 mg	Phosphorus	60.4 mg
/FIBER	0.8g	/Vitamin B-12	0.7 µg	Iron	1.3mg
/CHOLESTEROL	98.7 mg	/Vitamin B-6	1.1 mg	Calcium	18.1 mg
/PROTEIN	40.7g	/Niacin	21.2 mg	Vitamin-E	0.6mg
/SODIUM	367.4 mg	/Folate	16.5 µg	Vitamin-D	0.9µg

4. Twinkling Avocado Soup:

This soup is very easy to prepare and very tasty. If you are in a hurry then this is an ideal recipe for you to make in less than ten minutes.

Ingredients: - Almond milk (2 cups), - ripe avocados (2 medium), - cumin (½ teaspoon), - ground ginger (½ teaspoon), - garlic (1 clove, minced), and - salt (½ teaspoon or according to your taste).

Cooking details: Add all ingredients and mash avocados in a pan. Ideally, use an electric blender to mix all the ingredients well. Cook for an estimated 5 minutes and your soup is ready.

*Detailed nutritional breakup of the recipe:

Nutritional Value For Each Recipe:					
Twinkling Avocado Soup: Serving Size: 4					
/TOTAL CALORIES	797.5	/Vitamin-A	53.3 RE	Potassium	1200.4 mg
/TOTAL FAT	69.9	/Vitamin-	8.7	Zinc	4.1mg

	g	C	mg		
/SATURATED FAT	6.2g	/Thiamin (B-1)	0.3 mg	Magnesium	336.7 mg
/CARBO-HYDRATE	30.2g	/Riboflavin (B-2)	0.7 mg	Phosphorus	589.7 mg
/FIBER	17.6g	/Vitamin B-12	0.0 µg	Iron	4.7mg
/CHOLESTEROL	0.0 mg	/Vitamin B-6	0.4 mg	Calcium	259.2 mg
/PROTEIN	26.7g	/Niacin	5.6 mg	Vitamin-E	1.1mg
/SODIUM	329.1 mg	/Folate	83.4 µg	Vitamin-D	0.0µg

Helpful Items to have in the kitchen

- Raw honey (or agave syrup),

- Brown rice syrup,

- Pure maple syrup,

- Non-wheat flours (like rye, barley, spelt, rice, oat and quinoa),

- Lemons,

- Rice vinegar,

- Balsamic vinegar,

- Tarragon vinegar,

- Organic apple cider vinegar,

- Extra-virgin olive oil (only buy cold-pressed oil),

- Organic coconut oil for baking,

- Onions

- Garlic,

- Fresh vegetables,

- Brown rice,

 - Quinoa,

 - Oats,

- Amaranth,

- Other grains,

- Almond butter,

 - Pure maple syrup,

- Milk substitutes (like rice milk, almond milk, oat milk, soy milk),

- Beans & legumes both canned or dried,

- Dried spices & herbs (like basil, cumin, curry, oregano, thyme, nutmeg, garlic powder, sea salt, black pepper, cinnamon, turmeric, carob powder, mustard seeds, mustard powder, and many others),

- Filtered water,

 - Nuts and seeds,

- Fresh fruits,

- Large skillet (to fry vegetables),

- Large pot (mostly used for soups and sauces),

- Saucepan (for cooking grains and rice),

Chapter 13: Complementary Therapies

Ice T

Ice or cold therapy has been used for a long time as an effective home remedy for psoriatic arthritis. Ice has a cooling effect and at the same time it helps to numb the pain due to inflammation. It relaxes the muscles and joints and decreases the swelling around it. For cold treatment, ice packs can be used or in other cases bags of frozen vegetables wrapped in a towel can be made to eliminate pain. If the cold therapy is unbearable you may want to wrap it in a towel before applying. The total time of application should not exceed 3 minutes or so. Some researchers suggested that in order to avoid causing damage to skin and joints, apply ice packs for about 10 minutes then remove, then reapply for 10 minutes and again remove. When there is injury involving a muscle tendon, it is advised to run the ice across the entire length of the tendon, allowing it to enhance its mobility and healing. Keeping in mind the need of utilising ice packs, some pharmacies do carry frozen bags of beans or pellets that can be used specifically for swollen joints.

Fish Oil Supplements

Fish oil supplements contain the essential omega-3 fatty acids. There are three types of essential omega 3 fatty acids: alpha linolenic acid, eicosapentaenoic acid and docosahexaenoic acid. These omega-3 are potent anti-inflammatory and anti-oxidant agents. Omega 3 fatty acids inhibit the conversion of fatty acids to prostaglandins and leukotrienes in the body. Therefore, it is responsible for decreasing pain and inflammation. They help to remove the free radicals from the body, thereby minimising the injury related to the harmful substances in the body. Studies have shown that people who suffer from rheumatoid or psoriatic arthritis tend to get flare ups due to the constant, on-going inflammation within their bodies. So, omega 3 substances, especially fish oil supplements, help to decrease the inflammation around their joints thereby reducing the joint stiffness. For psoriatic arthritis 2g of EPA/DHA three times daily is the recommended dose. Other forms of fish oil may be found in salmon, mackerel, tuna and cod. Some studies suggest restricting the fish oil intake in pregnant women to no more than 8 ounces of tuna in a month. It has been recommended so as to keep the mercury levels in check without causing a significant increase in its level, which proves to be harmful for their baby. Also, it is advisable to avoid mackerel during pregnancy. You may find fish oil supplements over-the-counter. Caution must be sought so it is better to discuss your options with your doctor before starting any supplementations.

Avo-Kale Arthritis Arrester

Put kale with lime, salt and a few other vegetables like olives, garlic, carrot, parsley and black pepper. You may add all these ingredients in a large bowl, sprinkle some salt and leave it for some time. After this, transfer the kale into another bowl and squeeze some lime over it, making sure the lime is thoroughly mixed with it. From there on you may add avocado while slightly tossing the mixture. Add the rest of the ingredients in the remaining kale along with garlic and cashews. Sprinkle in some parsley, pepper and keep tossing it. You may add more seasonings or ingredients according to your own taste. Serve and enjoy this rich blend of vegetables to help in fighting off the inflammation.

These bright and green vegetables are a source of vital vitamins and minerals that help to get rid of harmful substances in the body. They are enriched with anti-oxidants, flavonoids and carotenoids. These are quite beneficial for patients with psoriatic arthritis. The avocado contains essential oils called the 'unsaponifiable fractions' that decrease pain and inflammation seen in cases of osteoarthritis and other joint diseases.

RICE: Rest, Ice, Compression, Elevation

This treatment is used to enhance the body's healing power and involves relaxing the tendons, muscles and joints. Usually, this therapy is started in those cases where there has been an acute injury or trauma to the body. It can be easily used for any area/part like the arms, knees and legs. It involves having a cloth, an ice pack, pillows and elastic wrap that may be optional. Instead of an ice pack, you may use a bag of frozen vegetables or peas; whatever is easily available. First of all, you would have to wet the cloth under the tap. Then dry it a little and wrap it around the ice pack, applying it directly to the sore site of injury. A pillow can be used as a means of supporting the injured part by placing it beneath it. It helps to give enough leverage to appropriately align the injured area so that there is minimal movement required.

At times, it is necessary to keep the injured part at a level above the heart so that it makes the circulation flow at a faster rate. After ten minutes, you may remove the ice pack and then let the injured part settle for about ten minutes. Repeat this procedure by placing the ice pack again for another ten minutes and then removing it. The elastic wrap can be of use by stabilising the joints, usually in cases where the injury is done to the ankle, knee joint or wrist so as to make it more stable and minimising range of the movements.

The basic technique is to start wrapping the joint a few inches from below it and wind until you reach a few inches above the joint. Care must be taken while wrapping the joint so that the blood circulation is not impeded as it could lead to severe tissue damage. You may check the looseness of the elastic wrap by sliding a finger or two under it. You may feel the need to repeat this procedure for about three days continuously. The mechanism behind this treatment is to allow the joints to rest in order for it to heal. The cold part helps to relieve pain by numbing the nerves and also decreases the swelling and inflammation around the joint. Pillow elevation is essential as it makes the circulation better and the flow of fluids that have been lost in injury can be reabsorbed returning it to the injured tissue. Wrapping the joint is needed so that some amount of compression is made necessary so you do not stretch or put undue pressure on the injured part. It reduces pain and inflammation as well. A study conducted by the British Journal of Sports medicine in the year 2006 proved that icing on for ten minutes and ten minutes off on the injured joints in people with sprained ankles had better results than people who had iced their joints straight for twenty minutes without any intervals. This can be dangerous as it leads to tissue necrosis due to excessive cold, stopping the blood circulation and resulting in tissue death.

Turmeric-Ginger Inflammation Fighter

In some patients of psoriatic arthritis, turmeric, which is a herb, has been found to reduce flare-ups. Turmeric is a herb in the ginger family and along with ginger it helps to control the inflammatory processes within the body. According to the National Psoriasis Foundation, turmeric and ginger both carry anti-inflammatory properties. You may even find it over-the-counter in the form of a supplement. Alternatively you can mix turmeric, ginger, onion, chicken stock, broccoli, carrots, cumin, red bell pepper, mushrooms, tofu and black pepper.

All the vegetables can either be sautéed or cooked over the skillet as per your requirements and taste. All these green leafy vegetables are considered to be full of anti-oxidants. Ginger and turmeric curry further enhance the anti-inflammatory and analgesic actions targeting the inflammatory portions in the body. They help to serve as a good source of all the vitally essential vitamins and minerals as well. It is always better to start after discussing such options with your doctor, as they may advise you to take the correct dosage for treatment. Some physicians say that turmeric has a mild effect on the immune system so it should not be expected to have a major impact on psoriatic arthritis. Keeping this in mind, some people have gained advantage from the continuous use of turmeric. A study conducted for a continuous period of three months showed that using 250 milligrams of ginger about four times a day could help to diminish pain especially in cases of osteoarthritis.

Muscle-Boosting Beet and Tart Cherry Tonic

It is a blended mixture of cherries and beetroot along with apples and ice cubes. This drink is useful before exercising due to the fact that it contains a lot of important anti-oxidants and anti-inflammatory agents. Cherries are vital to prevent muscle weakness and it can significantly help to reduce muscle problems that may occur after a workout. Some trials showed the results of people using cherry juice compared to a placebo juice every day for five day before running. After the workout, they drank cherry juice for two straight days. It had tremendous results in improving muscle weakness and showed an increase in the improvement of their joints and muscles. Beet juice is another favourite of the researchers, as it has been shown to efficiently improve muscle strength. There was also an enhanced supply of oxygen to the muscles, which proved its efficacy.

The athletes who were using beet juice had good results in their performance and vastly enhanced their muscle power. But, unfortunately there was a downside to using such juices; a decrease in the blood pressure was noted. Although the side effect was not significant, it was considered to be beneficial in some cases. Another theory that was postulated attributes to the daily consumption of about 45 cherries. This led to the fact that people who ate cherries everyday have a better response to the body's inflammatory response, as it tends to decrease the blood levels of such inflammatory chemicals. A study also showed that people who suffered from gout benefitted from eating cherries every day.

Açai Smoothie

Acai is a naturally occurring berry. It comes from a palm tree that grows in the Amazon in various parts of Central and South America. Some say that it contains anti-oxidants that help to fight off inflammation. Anti-oxidants are substances that tackle the free radicals that are harmful to different cells of the body. In this way, antioxidants decrease inflammation. Patients with psoriatic arthritis have pain due to joint inflammation and stiffness. Acai berry smoothies made from acai berries, bananas, strawberries, almonds and yogurt can eliminate these inflammatory mediator cells and improve joint health.

Acupuncture

Acupuncture is one of the oldest fields of science that deals with pins and needles. It has been proven beneficial in almost all types of arthritis be it rheumatoid, osteoarthritis or psoriatic arthritis. Studies have shown that acupuncture may not be helpful to a huge extent. They may be able to help a bit if not more as it has little association with the immune system. In psoriatic arthritis, as the immune system is hugely affected, acupuncture does not decrease the inflammatory processes but helps to reduce pain. For best results, acupuncture is advisable for isolated areas and not for the whole body.

Anti-Inflammatory Pineapple-Ginger Salsa

Pineapple and ginger salsa is easy to make and has a lot of benefits. All you need is pineapple and fresh ginger mixed with some lemon juice. Mix these ingredients in the blender and enjoy your pineapple ginger salsa. Pineapple and ginger are potent anti-inflammatory agents, as they contain enzymes called bromelain. This helps in eliminating pain and reduces inflammation. Research studies have indicated that bromelain along with turmeric is a powerful anti-inflammatory agent. Pineapple contains vitamin C, which helps to minimise oxidation reactions responsible for injury to the body. Ginger is an effective analgesic as well. During flare-ups of psoriatic arthritis, this unique combination of pineapple and ginger can decrease the pain and inflammation around the joints. Not only in cases of psoriatic arthritis. For people with osteoarthritis, ginger and pineapple salsa proved to relieve pain.

Herbal Pain-Relieving Poultice

Poultice is a unique mixture of various herbs. It contains aloe vera gel, olive oil, turmeric, ginger and cayenne pepper. It is blended in a bowl until its consistency is that of a paste. During a painful episode it is applied and later on washed with soap and water. Aloe vera is an anti-inflammatory and known to relieve pain. Olive oil is a powerful emollient that has been proved in random studies to be superior to some other analgesic ointments. Whereas ginger and turmeric are traditional herbs mostly found in the Indian part of the world. These two herbs are famous for minimising and eradicating pain and inflammation. Using these herbs for local application has been of great value. Cayenne pepper contains capsaicin and is a counter irritant. You may feel some burning sensation on first application but later on it will calm down the irritated nerves and soothe the sore muscles, thereby relieving pain in cases of psoriatic arthritis, rheumatoid arthritis, body aches and osteoarthritis. You should talk to your doctor before starting any herbal treatment, as you may end up having some allergic reaction.

Willow bark

Willow bark is a herb that has a similar effect to aspirin. A study that was conducted in the year 2001 showed the effect of willow bark compared to a 240mg dose of aspirin. It is difficult to confirm its benefits in patients with psoriatic arthritis, as studies are still controversial.

Lifestyle Tips & Modifications

Consider Magnets:

In some patients, the use of magnets helped to reduce pain in their joints. In cases of osteoarthritis and other joint diseases, wearing magnets has decreased the pain to a huge extent. Magnets in the form of bracelets, necklaces and pads are easily available on the market. Studies postulated that these magnets help to strengthen the natural magnetic field of the body. The body reacts to the electromagnetic fields around it in a positive manner. An example of it can be derived from the fact that when a muscle contraction occurs it induces signals from the nervous system that are strongly linked to the magnetic activity. There is still little evidence behind the science and how magnets interact with the body; further research is still needed to understand the mechanics of magnetic fields better. No harm has been observed; hence it is worth giving it a try at least once if not twice.

Stretch three times a week:

A few simple stretching exercises can help to improve joint functions. Stretching exercises help muscles to regain their full power and also help to reduce joint stiffness and soreness due to exercise. One problem that may be faced by patients with psoriatic arthritis is their joint laxity and range of motion, which should be kept in mind before such exercises. It is advised to do stretching exercises at least three times a week in order to maintain the functional status of the joints. Doing such stretching movements can help to minimise the risk of injury to the joints. However, in most cases running is not advised as it leads to a higher risk of injury and stress to the joints. Running at a higher pace and twisting motions can cause joint related damage worsening arthritis.

Castor oil pack:

Natural home remedies include various treatments; amongst them is using castor oil packs. Castor oil is an important oil that not only provides the emollient character but also helps to heal the wounds. You may use castor oil in addition to peppermint oil or ginger oil. Evidence through different studies has shown that using castor oil in massaging aids improves joint movements and significantly decreases the painful crisis during flare-ups. The technique is to massage the joints by applying castor oil around it rather than using it directly over the joints. Even in some cases it showed that if castor oil is applied and left overnight it leads to tremendous results.

Listen to your body:

It is essential and vital to do all the exercises according to your body's requirements. You may feel weak during the flare-ups, which make you unable to perform your daily activities. During such an episode it is important to seek help from your family and friends to help you cope up with the disease. If you do not find the strength to follow your daily exercise routine or do yoga during some day of the week, you should take rest and relax. This in turn will help you to start off with a better routine the very next day. It is not advised to push yourself through even if you do not have the power to work through a tough day. For example, during an episode of pain and joint inflammation, you may want to use an assistive devise to help you open the bottles, jars or doors for you so that you do not strain your fingers or hands. You may even want to avoid lifting heavy objects to minimise the joint damage to your back.

Sleeping at night assists your body to fight the fatigue and various inflammatory processes. So, it is very important to get a good night's sleep or a small nap in the afternoon. For a good sleep, you may want to set a pattern like going to bed during the same time every night or making a habit or taking a short nap during the afternoon. This helps you to wake up at the same time in the morning, making enough time for morning exercises. If due to some reason you have trouble sleeping, a warm bath may help to soothe your pain thereby facilitating sleep. Another tip that may benefit you is just to relax during your busy day by keeping your feet up for few minutes and listening to your favourite music or reading your favourite book.

Traveling Tips:

It can be a challenge to travel, especially if you are suffering from arthritis of any type. In order to travel daily or far and wide you may need to plan ahead and keep in mind the various scenarios that you can get stuck in during your travel. Day-to-day travel like driving your own car can be discussed with your therapist. There are many exercises that can be helpful in accommodating your different needs that can help you to tackle your car troubles. Preparing your car with adequate equipment is important, making modifications or searching for a car to cater to your comfort should be your first priority. As safety is the priority, comfort should also be looked upon while selecting a car for yourself. There are specialists that can teach you about your car as well as aid you with your driving techniques so that you may feel safe while handling the vehicle. Simple tips like adjusting your seat can prove to be useful. You may add a cover to the steering wheel so as to minimise the stress on your fingers and wrists, providing you with a smooth steering angle. Changing the interior of the car to a much more comfortable one can help to reduce joint related stress. For example, you may change the back seat of your car and place a beaded seat cover that will allow you to roll in and out of your seat, thereby minimising friction. The interior of the car can be changed to easy sliding objects, that way less pressure is applied to use them. Using gloves while driving will also reduce the pressure and assist to getting a nicer grip of the steering wheel.

Before driving you may do some warm up exercises, especially if it is going to be a long distance travel. It is important for people with psoriatic arthritis to move every two hours in order to keep their joints mobile and prevent joint stiffness. Hence, it is strongly advised to take breaks and stretch so that at the end of a long trip there is less pain and flexibility remains intact. Additional tips may include:

Carrying ice packs, hot packs, ice wraps, splints or pillows for your head or neck.

Managing your medication, which you may require in cases of an attack of pain.

Your prescription in order to get a refill from a nearby pharmacy, when required.

Eating healthily and drinking a lot of water so as to be thoroughly hydrated.

Avoiding any unhealthy or fried foods, as that can slow down your metabolism, making you sluggish and lethargic.

Keeping the important documents like insurance papers and medical IDs just in case of an emergency.

While traveling via the airport, book a flight that would be non-stop so that you would not have to leave the plane and go through additional security checking. At the airport, security checking is a major issue due to the amount of prescribed medications as well as handling your own luggage. It is thought to be wise to travel light and with as little baggage as possible. Asking for assistance can be done in cases where it seems difficult to carry your own luggage. In some cases, you may speak to the concerned authorities about your disability or medical condition that can be affected by the screening process. The scanners and body imaging equipment can be troublesome, especially if you have joint replacements or sensitive joints. Therefore, it is important to inform the airport's security personnel about the difficulties that you might face so as to gain assistance and help you travel with ease. Before reaching your destination, it would be suitable to inquire about the area that you might be living in or visiting. This way you would be well prepared about the surroundings and its weather, if they have a pool, beach or exercising centres etc. Planning your stay and having know-how about the means of transport is necessary.

Upon your arrival, inspect your room and its surroundings. If stairs are a problem for you, then you may ask for changes accordingly to help you have a comfortable stay. As people with psoriatic arthritis use medications that suppress their immune system, it makes them vulnerable to a lot of different infections. It is important to carry medications in your luggage for your trip. You may talk to your doctor about the immunisations that can help you prevent the diseases found in the place you will be travelling to. All in all, your condition should not stop you from traveling. It may need a bit of planning before you decide to travel but if you are prepared it is definite that you will end up enjoying your trip.

Mild Yoga:

Yoga is a form of exercise that includes mind and body relaxation. It consists of a variety of steps that help to control the body by doing breathing, stretching and strengthening exercises. Yoga also aids in improving the sleep routine and enhances the mood. In people suffering from psoriatic arthritis, yoga helps to eliminate joint pain and improves the range of motion. It is recommended to practice yoga for about 15-20 minutes daily to achieve the desired response. Be sure to check for the appropriate instructor and class so that the program supports your needs and understands the type of exercise best suited for you.

Aloe Vera:

Psoriatic arthritis is a lifelong disease that can be triggered by external factors. By limiting exposure to such triggers, episodes of flare-ups can be minimised. Aloe vera has potent anti-bacterial and anti-inflammatory properties so it is effective when in the form of gels or creams for the treatment of psoriatic arthritis. When applied topically, aloe vera has a cooling effect and it helps to reduce redness, swelling and pain when used regularly. Studies have postulated that patients who constantly use aloe vera for their joints have a better result and improvement in their joint mobility compared to those using topical steroids. The usual dose is local application is three to four times daily to achieve maximum results. Some studies reported aloe vera's use orally for the treatment of various other diseases such as ulcerative colitis, hepatitis and even cancer. So it can be safely said that aloe vera minimises the inflammation that leads to psoriasis outbreaks responsible for joint damage. It promotes collagen and elastin repair along with some other important vitamins boosts body health.

Chinese Herbs:

Chinese herbs have been found useful in treating the symptoms related to psoriatic arthritis. Some plant extracts like the Tripterygium wilfordii are thought to have some anti-inflammatory properties. A study that was conducted by the National Institutes of Health concluded that patients who were taking this plant herb had better outcomes compared to the patients who were taking non-steroidal anti-inflammatory drugs. This effect has been specially attributed to a drug azuflidine and those taking steroids.

Spa Treatments:

People since ancient times have tried to relax by using various methods; one of them being bathing. For people with psoriatic arthritis. especially after a long strenuous work out, it may prove to be very useful. Some people like to use Epsom salts or essential oils in their bathing routine. You may combine the salt and essential oils like rosemary, cypress, ginger or cedar wood oil and add it to a tub of warm water. Such techniques have a soothing and calming effect on the body. It reduces the soreness of the muscles and relieves the joint aches as well. Epsom salts have been used to treat muscle aches for quite some time. They contain magnesium sulphate which causes the muscles to relax. In some studies a mixture of calcium, sulphate and magnesium salts have known to reduce pain in many patients, especially those who are suffering from different types of arthritis. Since there are not many on-going studies supporting the use of such herbs, it is hard to determine the extent of its effectiveness. Based on their use since ancient times, it is not a loss to try it for some time. An alternative to long baths can be a hot shower that is an easy and quick way to relieve from muscle soreness and aches.

Balneotherapy:

Balneotherapy is a treatment that includes bathing in naturally occurring heated mineral water. It has been very effective for various diseases. It has been linked to spa therapies as well as water baths, mineral baths, mud baths and others. In balneotherapy, a person spends time in a naturally occurring thermal mineral water or in a heated pool containing different minerals. Such minerals may include sodium, bicarbonate, magnesium, sulphur and others. The mechanism of balneotherapy is that it helps to reduce the inflammatory processes, hence decreasing pain and affecting the immune system. It has been said to reduce pain and improve the functional status of the psoriatic joints if used over a period of three months. Due to its short-term effects, a lot of scientists still disagree upon the advantages of balneotherapy. However, it is advised to take sulphur and Dead Sea minerals baths as it has profound effects on the joints, improving the life quality of the patients. A study showed that balneotherapy had significantly improved the mobility in active joints and reduced the tender joints in both males and females. Further researches are required to correctly assess the effect of balneotherapy with psoriatic arthritis.

Tai chi:

As we know, exercise is important for patients with psoriatic arthritis, and one form is tai chi. Tai chi is a Chinese form of martial arts. It is an old form of martial arts that means supreme ultimate fist. In recent times it has gotten popular due to its easy-to-do steps. It has many components, which include stretching, slow focused exercising moves and deep breathing. This is an excellent combination that helps to ease the pain and at the same time increasing the flexibility of the joints. You may need to contact a martial arts school that can help you learn it the correct way. There are hundreds of long and short moves that do not involve heavy or strenuous moves. The steps may include standing poses and simple arm movements. It focuses on the posture, conscious levels and movement stability.

Hence, little to no strength is required to perform Tai chi. As little as ten or twelve moves can be adjusted, depending on the requirements of your body. Hence it makes Tai chi an easy form of exercise that can be adapted by people with all levels of functional abilities. Tai chi can be done at home, in the park or anywhere else, making it more suitable for all ages and groups. It can even be done in water, no additional equipment is required and that is an additional benefit of learning Tai chi. According to the American college of rheumatology, Tai chi is included as the non-drug therapy for psoriatic arthritis patients.

Scientific evidence showed that Tai chi helps to reduce the pain associated with psoriatic arthritis. It helps to improve the functional capacity to perform daily activities. Apart from all the other benefits, Tai chi has helped in improving self-esteem and motivation, causing a significant reduction in the level of anxiety and depression.

Exercise:

It is quite hard for a person with psoriatic arthritis to exercise, especially when they are going to a painful episode. When such an incident occurs when your joints are stiff and pain does not go away, you may find it hard to exercise, but that's okay! In other days when the pain is relatively less you may be in a better position to exercise. Exercise helps to strengthen the muscles and increases the flexibility of the joints. Therefore it is necessary to work out at least 10 to 20 minutes daily to regain the muscle power and joint stability. Another alternative to daily workouts is exercising in a pool. The water in the pool helps to build muscle strength and is less stressful for your joints. As exercise is important, the pool water will support your joints without increasing the inflammatory process or wear and tear. Exercising is also known to reduce weight and maintain your own weight so that there is no additional pressure on your major weight bearing joints. Other exercises can be discussed with your physiotherapist depending on your body's requirements, keeping in mind to exercise the joints in their range of motion.

Chapter 14: 25 Best & Easy Coping Steps for PA Patients:

A very common situation that a lot of patients can come across during the initial period of their illness is how to start dealing with their illness and related symptoms. If you have read the book in detail, you have been well informed about psoriatic arthritis. We have also comprehensibly covered the dietary section to allow readers to fight against their demons on a daily basis. Still, both as a reader and as a patient you should now start to work on a specific step-by-step program to make sure that you or your loved ones are on the right track to overcoming psoriatic arthritis and related complications. Experts in rheumatology from around the world have designed various coping strategies and programs to counter this devil aggressively. However, I have chosen a 25-step strategy for the readers as I have found these guidelines to be the most comprehensive among the rest.

25 Top PA Coping Steps:

PA symptoms are inevitable and require few lifestyle changes to control. The following 25 steps are provided to patients looking to take charge of their illness. These 25 steps will allow you to cope with PA long-term.

*** Step 1**: *Conquest Psoriasis & Psoriatic Arthritis*:

Clearly, Psoriatic arthritis and psoriasis are most challenging when it comes to coping with the related symptoms. Nevertheless, illnesses are never out of control until we are no longer eager to fight back. Every sufferer should start by learning about the illness. Psoriatic arthritis (PA) is an autoimmune disease and certainly manageable. Motivate yourself and start implementing the following plan in your life to achieve the best results. It will help you and your close ones over a long period. The program is designed to help you manage your symptoms in the best possible manner. The following guidelines will allow you to soothe and subdue disturbing symptoms, encourage your confidence and promote coping abilities.

Life is precious and you only get one chance to make it right. I have always believed in "God helps those who help themselves".

*** Step 2**: *Start with Weight Loss*:

Obesity/being overweight is a top health concern around the globe, regardless of origin, age and gender. Obesity/being overweight can impose a serious impact on most life-threatening illnesses and symptoms. Obesity has a considerable impact on all of the following chronic illnesses:

- Diabetes,

- Heart-related disorders,

- Cancer,

- Infertility,

- Joint pain,

- Ulcers,

- Skin disorders, and

– Gallstones.

Psoriatic arthritis and weight are mostly inter-connected, especially with increased joint pain and inflammation. More weight can result in increased pressure on joints and bones. Added pressure always results in further pain and accelerates the disintegration of tendons and bones at crucial points. The joints of the knees and ankles are prime examples of added pressure related to obesity. If you can successfully manage to reduce and maintain a healthy weight then you can definitely manage pain, inflammation and related symptoms of Psoriatic arthritis.

Weight Loss: Natural Tips for Amazing Results:

Weight loss can be easy to achieve but sometimes we are not ready to accept it. We have many reasons to do so. Reasons like we know that we cannot manage some lifestyle changes essential for weight loss. For example, managing our eating habits, our daily physical routine and our sleep patterns is difficult. Everyone knows that such lifestyle adjustments can certainly enable us to lose and maintain a healthy weight. Personal fitness trainers and nutritionists from around the world have contributed immensely to help psoriatic arthritis patients shed extra pounds. Without making it too complex for the readers, let's read some relatively easier and doable things. Follow this popular and affective 5-tip solution for easy weight loss and you will see remarkable results in no time.

- Weight Loss Tip #1: Green Tea: Green tea is gaining huge popularity is weigh loss market.

- Weight Loss Tip #2: Limit Fructose Intake: Limiting fructose intake on a daily basis is a vital step for beginners.

- Weight Loss Tip #3: Eat Organic: Avoiding processed food and shifting to organic food items can help shed unwanted pounds.

- Weight Loss Tip #4: Workout at Home: Going regularly to the gym can be very difficult for most. Devote some time to small exercises at home and you will notice remarkable change within weeks.

- Weight Loss Tip #5: Herbs & Spices: Herbs and spices are very famous in Asian and Mediterranean regions. Peppers, ginger, garlic, turmeric, and many more are known to be effective in controlling fat deposits in abdominal region.

*** Step 3**: *Sunlight: A blessing of Nature*:

Over the centuries, humans have learned well to utilise natural resources. Some natural resources are inevitable but very beneficial for mankind, like the sun. Sunlight is a great source of energy, not only mechanically but also for individuals. Our bones and skin can absorb healthy nutrients like vitamin D and vitamin K from the sunlight. Some patients' data has provided support to the idea that spending a few minutes every day under sunlight can show improvement in psoriasis and psoriatic arthritis. Even if there is no scientific data available, exposing your skin to sunlight for a little while is harmless.

* Step 4: *Protect Your Scalp:*

Several pharmaceutical companies are now manufacturing coal-tar shampoos, sprays, soaps, gels and hand lotions. Such products can reduce skin irritation. These products are vital for psoriasis and psoriatic arthritis patients.

* Step 5: *Keep Yourself & Your Joints Fit*:

You can start with a simple exercise plan that you can later take to advance level. Exercise will allow movement necessary to keep your body going. Exercise is also ideal to control and prevent all types of joint-related problems. Start with 5 minutes a day to 30 minutes. Gradually increase your duration and intensity to avoid any potential hazards.

* Step 6: *Manage time for Manicures*:

Skin irritation is very common in Psoriatic arthritis. Try and manage regular manicures for a better and less irritated skin. Manicures will keep your skin and nails clean to provide soothing affects.

* Step 7: *Cosmetic Try-outs*:

As already told, there are multiple products available to limit PA symptoms. Females can also try cosmetic products that can help them reduce disturbing feelings. Ideally, use fragrance free, non-comedogenic and non-acnegenic products. Makeup will also allow visual beauty and self-confidence.

* Step 8: *Take Baths Appropriately*:

Spending too much or too little time in the shower is not a good idea, especially when you are suffering from skin and joint-related problems. Ask your rheumatologist for the exact time you should be spending in the shower. A rheumatologist will guide you properly after analysing your skin and joint condition.

Furthermore, use moisturisers on a regular basis to keep your skin healthy.

Step 9: *Eating the Perfect Way*:

We have discussed the ups and downs of PA in the perspective of obese, overweight and unhealthy individuals. Whatever the case may be, a healthy diet is always significant to counter inflammatory symptoms. A comprehensive diet plan with amazingly delicious recipes is included in this book for you. Refer to the diet and PA section of the book.

Step 10: Stress Management:

A stressed mind and body both are vulnerable to health complications. A peaceful mind and a healthy body are inevitable to overcome PA complications. Make it your priority; it will prove to be a blessing in disguise. Allow your mind and body to relax and avoid stressful situations both physically and mentally.

Step 11: Junk food is bad for your PA:

About 70 per cent of our young population is shifted to junk food. Junk food is mostly rich in sugar, oil and gluten. It can be very bad for individuals who have a tendency towards PA. Avoid junk food and try to consume foods rich in nutrients and fibre. Spinach, olive oil, dates and nuts are best eating options for all age groups.

Step 12: Alcohol & Substance abuse:

Humans have adapted to some social and personal habits that are solely against our physical and mental growth. Drug addiction and alcoholism can null and void all efforts to fight against PA.

Step 13: Smoking is a bad habit:

Smoking is another bad habit. It may cause a PA patient serious exhaustion during exercise. If quitting is not an option then make sure to limit nicotine-rich items and alcohol. Also, spread this message to everyone you love and know.

*** Step 14***: ***Meditation: Body & Mind Relaxation Technique***:

Meditate your mind and body to a point of relaxation and optimal physical health. You can manage some time on a daily basis to meditate and try to take control of your illness rather than allowing it to control you. PA or any other illness requires comprehensive treatment and a peaceful mental approach. Meditation is a great way to achieve both simultaneously.

*** Step 15***: ***Start Taking Prescriptions***:

You can never be on your own to cope with PA. Professional advice and medications are a huge support for every PA patient. PA can reach a point of unbearable pain and discomfort and medication is certainly a good option. Advancements in the field of pharmacology are allowing for the better treatment of PA with medications. Nonetheless, some medications used for PA are also associated with several adverse effects if used long-term or in high doses.

*** Step 16***: ***Choose Daily Household Items Wisely***:

It is very important that you understand the importance of your daily lifestyle choices. For example, a housewife suffering from PA should avoid buying heavy kitchen items. Make sure to avoid heavy weight lifting at all costs. It may lead to increased or even intolerable pain.

*** Step 17***: ***Pick The Right Clothing***:

Dress properly to cover your body from sunlight if you are suffering from skin-related PA symptoms. Exposure to sunlight can be good but extended exposure can increase irritation and red patches.

*** Step 18***: ***Perfumes & Deodorants***:

Be careful while choosing your cosmetic products, perfumes and deodorants. All these are very common in use. Make sure that all your daily use products including soap are allergen free.

*** Step 19***: ***Alternative Therapies***:

Multiple alternative therapies are available to cope with several chronic illnesses. PA symptoms, mainly pain, can be treated and reduced with alternative therapies like yoga. Yoga is famous for weight loss, physical fitness and mental relaxation. So, yoga can be a better option to adopt for PA.

* Step 20: Cotton & Silk:

Choosing the right fabric is very important. Some fabrics can be very irritating to the skin. Ideally, either use soft cotton or silk fabrics. Additionally, some colours are better than others. Avoid wearing black and other dark colours. Light colours can also provide a soothing effect.

* Step 21: Physiotherapy & Psychotherapy:

If you ever feel that your body and mind are unable to take the toll of the disease then you can opt for both physiotherapy and psychotherapy.

* Step 22: Social Interactions:

Creating a group of people facing a similar disease is a good idea. Share your personal experiences and information with others to explore new possibilities for treatment and prevention. Expressing emotions can also provide a psychological boost.

* Step 23: Side effects of Medications for PA:

If your PA symptoms have flared-up then you must be on medications. However, you must use medications only in prescribed doses because several complications can take place with overdosing on PA-medications.

Examples of Potential Disorders:

- Acute renal failure,
- Headache,
- Rash,
- Nervousness,
- Dry mouth and dry eyes,
- Tinnitus,

- Nausea,
- Heartburn,
- Abdominal cramping,
- Decrease appetite,
- Oedema,
- Dizziness,
- Fluid retention,
- Allergic reactions,
- Gastric or duodenal ulcer,
- Raised liver enzymes,
- Neutropenia,
- Agranulocytosis,
- Thrombocytopenia,
- Bronchospasm or asthma,
- Stevens
- Johnson syndrome.

Step 24: Omega 3 Fatty acids:

Fish, fish oils and other fish products can play a significant role in joint rehabilitation and the reduction of inflammation in joints. Seafood like fish are rich in omega 3 fatty acids that are vital for joint and skin restructuring.

Step 25: Travel & Tourism:

A change of location, atmosphere and temperature may result in positive feelings and a reduction of symptoms. Travelling around can also give you hope to fight PA symptoms and live a healthier life.

Chapter 15: Top Supplements for Psoriatic Arthritis

Using supplements can be an effective way of coping with PA symptoms, especially for pain, inflammation and bone strength.

Micronutrients are required to carry out fundamental functions in our body. Major organs in the human body require nutrients to perform effectively. Humans consume different foods to absorb these nutrients like vitamins and minerals. Deficiency of any of these nutrients (mainly vitamin-A, vitamin-D, vitamin-C, Zinc, Calcium, Copper, Iron and Potassium) can result in serious health – mental and physical - complications. Using supplements to cover potential deficiencies can be very helpful.

The supplement industry has grown immensely. You can easily find good multivitamins and herbal supplements from local markets. Most of us are well informed about basic nutrients but rarely realise the importance of herbs and other nutrients to cope with PA symptoms. We have tried to include some quality information from most reputable sources to ensure support on a larger scale to the readers.

The role and mechanism of some basic nutrients, micronutrients and herbs (plants) in Psoriatic Arthritis is explained below:

Antioxidants

We are lucky to have antioxidants available to us in the form of herbs like acai berry, goji berry, mangosteen, Hawaiian noni and pomegranate, as well as in the form of micronutrients like vitamin-C, vitamin-A and vitamin-E. Antioxidants are vital in fighting off the free radicals formed due to the breakdown of various metabolic processes. Our body undergoes stress during all the biologic processes. In order to keep up with the free radicals and to minimise injury to the body, antioxidant supplementation is required on daily basis.

Antioxidants can play a part in optimising health in PA patients by promoting the body's metabolic functions and help the body to cope on its own. It also helps to minimise free-radical injury so that harmful toxins are eliminated and are not accumulated in the body. Most of the toxins are produced by pollution, smoking, radiation, sunlight and smoking, which in turn lead to increased production of free radicals.

Whenever there is an increase in oxidative stress in the body, gluthathione levels are depleted. Antioxidants can play a part in increasing the catalase and super oxide dismutase and gluthathione peroxidase levels. This results in a massive reduction of oxidative stress, minimising damage and oxidative injury to the healthy cells of the body. As a result of decreased oxidative damage, inflammatory mediators are reduced. Hence, Antioxidants acts as an anti-inflammatory agent.

Top dietary sources of antioxidants:

- Fruits,

- Vegetables,

- Berries,

- Carrots,

- Pecan,

- Plum,

- Black plum,

- Sweet cherry, and

 - Apples.

Hawaiian noni

Hawaiian Noni is an extract used in alternative medicine for its various benefits including anti-inflammatory, analgesic, anti-tumour, antibacterial, antiviral, hypotensive and as an immune enhancing agent. Consuming appropriate amounts of Hawaiian noni extract can be life changing for Psoriatic arthritis patients. It works by repairing cells of the body that are damaged and activates immune mediated responses.

Goji berry

Goji berry has been famous for its action on almost all the organs of the body. It helps to regulate sleep patterns, lowers blood pressure, lowers joint pain and inflammation, helps people with diabetes and age-related eye problems. It has a calming effect on the nervous system and improves the quality of sleep along with a relaxed mood. Again a healthy sleeping pattern is very important, even if you are a PA patient or not. A good amount of goji berry can be vital to support your body in coping with PA symptoms with improved health.

Resveratrol: Fat Reduction in PA Patients

Controlling and reducing body weight to a standard is crucial for PA patients to minimise the pressure on the joints and bones. Resveratrol can be used as an effective way of treating obesity and overweight problems. Resveratrol is known for its effect on lipid mobilisation, helping to reduce fat stores. It is a phytochemical that inhibits the differentiation of preadipocytes, stimulates lipolysis and induces apoptosis of existing adipocytes. These mechanisms further reduce adipose tissue mass in the body. Also, resveratrol increases fat breakdown in the mature adipocytes hence reducing fat formation in adipocytes.

Beta-sitosterol: An Exceptional Immune modulation

Ideally, a supplement should be such a chemical that has numerous benefits, and works to improve many aspects of the body's physiology. Beta-sitosterol does exactly this and is therefore an exceptional nutritional option for everyone. Beta-sitosterol is a substance mainly found in plants (plant sterol) and is chemically similar to cholesterol in the human blood. Over the years, researchers have found multiple benefits of taking this chemical as a nutrient. Firstly, it has vital effects on the levels of certain lipids in the body and in this way reduces one of the major risks for cardiac disease. Then it has been implicated in the treatment of benign prostatic hyperplasia, a distressful disease of the prostate. Another area of use is in the prevention of male pattern baldness, a testosterone-mediated disease like BPH. Recently its use has been found in the treatment of breast cancer. Lastly, it has overall effects on improving immunity and health of the body. This health use can benefit PA patients hugely.

Immunity is a complex system consisting of a whole array of cells that are responsible for various defence mechanisms. Too much or too little activation leads to devastating effects of either autoimmune diseases destroying host cells immune deficiency leading to opportunistic infections. Psoriatic arthritis and other types of autoimmune diseases are few that are caused by a malfunction of our immune system. Therefore, a balance is needed to run the system. It has been found by researchers that beta-sitosterol is an excellent immune modulator. It helps in the production and proper maturation of T lymphocytes and NK cells that are central to fighting off infections. On the other hand, they stop abnormal antibody formation and spread. Hence, use of this chemical has been implicated in the treatment of numerous immune dysfunctions. Certainly, Beta-sitosterol can be equally effective for PA patients in neutralizing their pain and inflammation.

Dietary sources: It is found mainly in plant products such as;

- Fruits,

- Vegetables,

- Soybeans,

- Breads,

- Peanuts and

- Peanut products.

Goldenseal: Immune Stimulant

Goldenseal is a plant whose extract and powder has been used in medicine for many decades. It has proved to be very effective in boosting and modulating our immunity responses. Macrophages are one of the main fighters of infection in our body, but when they start to do their work they release some substances that cause inflammation, which is responsible for the many negative symptoms of several diseases and infections. This extract stimulates the macrophages and fights diseases/infection but decreases the effects of those pro-inflammatory chemicals. It also regulates the immune response to the common viral and bacterial infections. It stimulates the immunity by working on the cytokines and decrease the inflammatory response. Therefore, taking Goldenseal as a supplement can ensure an adequate response to a wide number of autoimmune diseases including Psoriatic Arthritis.

Natural Amino Acids

Amino acids are essential as they are required for various metabolic processes in our body. They help to regulate energy stores and provide you with glucose so that you may meet your daily energy requirements efficiently.

Arginine is a natural α-amino acid and a pivotal building block in our body. It serves to play a very integral role in the body where it essentially helps and supports cell division and protein synthesis, being two of the most major bodily functions. The sufficient dietary intake or supplementation of arginine is needed to meet the daily requirements. High doses of proteins are required at stages where there is a loss and deficiency of proteins like pregnancy, periods of growth and childhood. It can be equally important for PA patients for bone and muscle health. Arginine readily contributes to improve capillary growth and muscles.

Arginine & Exercise for PA:

Arginine and other amino acids can help to effectively regulate hormones in the body. One such effect is seen of arginine on the growth hormone production. Exercise leads to the stimulation of the growth hormone and with L-arginine supplementation its response is gradually increased. Therefore, growth of cells is enhanced by a considerable margin. This phenomenon can be of the utmost importance for both young and adult PA patients.

Lean body mass in PA patients:

Ornithine and Arginine have a vital role in maintaining the body's metabolic functions. A study was conducted where two groups were evaluated, one using ornithine and arginine compared to the other one using a placebo agent. Daily supplementation of ornithine and arginine resulted in total strength and lean body mass. There was a significant increase in the strength of the individuals using arginine. The study concluded that arginine and ornithine not only helped to recover from daily stressors but it also enhanced recovery from chronic stress like conditions.

Glutamine, Arginine, Bovine colostrum & Ornithine

Glutamine, arginine, bovine colostrum and ornithine play an important role during physical stress. There is a constant need for proteins and energy, which may be supplied at short intervals. Bovine Colostrum supplementation in various trials concluded its use for 8 weeks, which may increase bone-free lean body mass in active men and women. Bovine colostrum promotes immune, growth and has antimicrobial activity that helps in the development of tissues and improves immune functions necessary in physical performance.

Major dietary sources of amino acids:

- Spinach,

 - Red meat,

- Nuts,

- Whole grains,

- Walnuts,

- Lentils,

- Seafood,

- Soy, and

– Eggs.

Liquorice

Liquorice is easily available in supplements and is a plant used for flavouring in foods, beverages and tobacco. Various medicinal uses have been suggested for liquorice, these including sore throat, bronchitis, cough, heartburn, osteoarthritis, psoriatic arthritis, liver disorders, malaria, tuberculosis and chronic fat syndrome. This herb has also been studied for its use in improving infertility in women when used in combination with other herbs. The liquorice herb has strong anti-inflammatory, antivirus, anti-ulcer and anti-carcinogen properties. It has been reviewed for its effect on tumour-like cells to inhibit their growth and proliferation. People have used Liquorice as a weight-reducing herb. High potency fibre complexes must be consumed in supplementation with appropriate amounts of liquorice providing you the best combination of herbs along with fibre.

Psyllium husk for PA patients

Regular use of Psyllium husk can be a life changing remedy for PA patients with a body weight on the higher side. Psyllium husk is effective for people suffering from obesity, high blood sugar levels and cholesterol disorders. Obesity is being overweight with a BMI of greater than 30. Obesity is associated with several chronic symptoms and disorders just like it can play a major role in increasing the severity of Psoriatic arthritis symptoms. Increased body weight can impose unwanted, painful stress on bones and joints in PA patients. Controlling body weight with Psyllium husk can benefit the human body in several ways, for instance obesity leading to high insulin levels by causing their resistance in the body. These high blood sugar levels tend to be a contributing factor causing Diabetes type II. A good glycaemia control is needed once diabetes is developed, otherwise iy may eventually cause cardiovascular disease like myocardial infarction, atherosclerosis and angina. Therefore, the desirable effect of fibres, especially psyllium husk helps to reduce body weight and satiety, on cholesterol, on fasting glycaemia and on blood pressure suggesting it to have an important role in prevention of various cardiac diseases.

Hyaluronic acid, Boswellia serrata & Methylsulphomethane

Inflammation is a physiological process in which the body reacts to the abnormal condition and informs the system of the body by giving manifestation such as redness, heating, loss of function and pain. Macrophages will accumulate at the site of inflammation and start cleaning the mess over there. They will start to remove the dead cells and start repairing of connective tissue by depositing proteins.

Function in Inflammation & Pain:

Joint is a fluid filled cavity that is filled by fluid that protects the bones to colloid. It is insulation between all the joints. In some diseases, the process of inflammation causes a decrease of production of this fluid that causes pain. Osteoarthritis and Psoriatic arthritis are the most common inflammation disorders of the joints and mostly women are affected with these two disorders. Studies have shown that hyaluronic acid, Boswellia serrata and Methylsulphomethane are effective in the treatment of joint pain and inflammation. Hyaluronic acid is injected in the knees of patients with severe disability problem. It not only improves the level of pain in joints by decreasing inflammation but also increases the function of joint.

Methylsulphomethane is present in sulphur mostly. It is found in onions, garlic, crucified vegetables, nuts, milk and egg in small amounts. It is used in the prevention and treatment of psoriatic arthritis and osteoarthritis. It is being proved that MSM is an anti-inflammatory agent that decreases the pain, swelling and improves the functional ability of joints.

121

The _Boswellia serrata_ tree is found in India mostly. Its glue is being used in joint inflammation. It decreases pain and swelling of the joints and increases the flexion of knee. It can help patients cover more distance during walking because of decrease of inflammation and pain.

Bromelain & Celadrin

Inflammation first increases the blood flow and then decreases it physiologically to prevent the loss of blood. Due to stasis and the decrease movement of the blood, platelets start to aggregate and can cause thrombophlebitis. It is serious, which should be addressed on time to prevent complications. Bromelain and celadrin both inhibit the platelets aggregation and have anti-thrombotic and fibrinolytic activity.

Bromelain is a crude extract of pineapples that is being used in the inhibition of platelet aggregation for so many years and it is very effective without side effects. It also has anti-inflammatory, anti-tumour, and anti-oedematous, and modulate the immune system.

Celadrin is made of special fats derived from bovine tallow oil. It works by covering all the membranes of the body and causes the restoration of fluids that cushion the bones and prevent inflammatory response. It inhibits the platelets' aggregation and helps to prevent thrombus formation.

Green-lipped mussel & Shark cartilage

All of the diseases of joints have a common denominator; that is the inflammation of the joint surfaces and space. The source of damage to the joint can be either wear and tear leading to degeneration like Osteoarthritis or can be autoimmune reactions like Psoriatic and Rheumatoid arthritis. Whatever the case may be the result is excessive and uncontrolled inflammation, which is a process involving the release of active chemicals into the joint space leading to fluid leak, redness, warmth and pain. This results in the inability to use the joint freely, mostly due to pain. This supplement is a scientific blend of natural ingredients that has an extremely potent anti-inflammatory action. Green-lipped mussel (a shellfish in New Zealand) and shark cartilage (dried and powdered cartilage of a shark) decreases the chemical mediators responsible for increasing capillary permeability and inflammation. This results in miraculous improvements in joint function and mobility.

Above was a quick overview of some effective ingredients easily accessible through supplements and can be consumed for considerable improvements in PA symptoms.

Suggested Studies

1. *Psoriatic Arthritis: New Insights for the Healthcare Professional*:

2011 Edition is a Scholarly Brief™ that delivers timely, authoritative, comprehensive, and specialised information about Psoriatic Arthritis in a concise format.

The editors have built Psoriatic Arthritis: New Insights for the Healthcare Professional: 2011 Edition on the vast information databases of Scholarly News.™ You can expect the information about Psoriatic Arthritis in this eBook to be deeper than what you can access anywhere else, as well as consistently reliable, authoritative, informed, and relevant. The content of Psoriatic Arthritis: New Insights for the Healthcare Professional: 2011 Edition has been produced by the world's leading scientists, engineers, analysts, research institutions, and companies. All of the content is from peer-reviewed sources, and all of it is written, assembled, and edited by the editors at Scholarly Editions™ and available exclusively from us. You now have a source you can cite with authority, confidence, and credibility.

2. *Natural Treatments for Psoriasis and Psoriatic Arthritis*:

15 April, 2014 by Jerome Aguilar.

Are You Ready to Find Out Everything You Need to Know About Psoriasis and Psoriatic Arthritis? Do You Suffer From the Itching and Scaling of Psoriasis? Or the Chronic Agony of Psoriatic Arthritis? If so you are not ALONE! A whopping three per cent of the world's population suffers from either condition! An incredible 56 million working hours are lost every year by psoriasis sufferers according to the National Psoriasis Foundation.

The drugs to manage psoriasis are expensive and have side effects! Although the disease is not fatal it can be so annoying you wish you were dead!

References

* The Anti-Inflammation Diet and Recipe Book BY Jessica k. Black

* Meals that Heal Inflammation by Julie Daniluk.

* The Everything Anti-Inflammation Diet Book by Karlyn Grimes.

* The Anti-Inflammatory Diet Plan by Robert M Fleischer.

* www.arthritistoday.org

* Genetic and Environmental Risk Factors for Psoriatic Arthritis among Patients with Psoriasis: Lihi Eder, University of Toronto, 2011.

* Immunological Studies of Psoriatic Arthritis: by Katrin Zipperlen, Memorial University of Newfoundland (Canada). 2008.

* New Therapeutic Targets in Rheumatoid Arthritis By Paul-Peter Tak.

 * Diagnostic Imaging of Musculoskeletal Diseases: A Systematic Approach: by Akbar Bonakdarpour, William R. Reinus, Jasvir S. Khurana. 2010.

* Compartments: How the Brightest, Best Trained, and Most Caring People Can Make Judgments That Are Completely and Utterly Wrong. Steven R. Feldman, 2009.

* Mapping Systemic Lupus Erythematosus and Psoriatic Arthritis in Greater Toronto Area Using Geographic Information Systems. Mustafa H. Al-Maini, University of Toronto (Canada), 2008.

* Imaging Strategies for the Knee: The human knee, with its complex anatomy and frequent disorders, undergoes radiologic examination more than any other joint. Imaging Strategies for the Knee organizes all of the relevant information clinicians need to

help them reach a sound diagnosis, accurately and efficiently. By Juergen Maeurer Thieme, 01-Jan-2011.

* Clinical Trials in Rheumatology, Volume 1 by Ruediger Mueller, Johannes von Kempis, 2012.

* Combined Scintigraphic and Radiographic Diagnosis of Bone and Joint Diseases,

 By Yong-Whee Bahk, H.N.Jr. Wagner, 2008.

* Taking Control of Your Psoriatic Arthritis: A Practical Guide to Treatments, Services and Lifestyle Choices, Paul Bird, Mona Marbani, Peter Nash, Peter Youssef, Judith Nguyen, Arthritis Australia, 2008.

* Autoimmune Diseases: Acute and Complex Situations: Munther A Khamashta, Manuel Ramos-Casals

* Radiological Features of Psoriatic Arthritis: Razaan Davis, University of Cape Town, 2011.

* Podiatry: A Psychological Approach: By Anne Mandy, Kevin Lucas, Janet McInnes, Jodie Lucas, 2011.

* Approach to Internal Medicine: A Resource Book for Clinical Practice By David Hui.

* Lecture Notes: Clinical Pharmacology and Therapeutics: By Gerard A. McKay, John L. Reid, Matthew R. Walters.

* Pediatric Rheumatology in Clinical Practice, 2011.

 By Patricia Woo, Ronald M. Laxer, David D. Sherry.

* Inflammation Nation: The First Clinically Proven Eating Plan to End Our Nation's Secret Epidemic. 2006. By Floyd H. Chilton

* Osteoimmunology: Interactions of the Immune and skeletal systems II By Yongwon Choi.

* The Journal of Rheumatology, Volume 35, Issue 4: Journal of Rheumatology Publishing Company, 2008.

* Osteoimmunology: Interactions of the Immune and Skeletal Systems edited by Joseph Lorenzo, Mark Horowitz, Yongwon Choi, Georg Schett, Hiroshi Takayanagi.

* Handbook of Pediatric Psychology, Fourth Edition, Edited by Michael C. Roberts, Ric G. Steele.

* Advances in TNF Family Research: Proceedings of the 12th International TNF Conference, 2009. By David Wallach, Andrew Kovalenko, Marc Feldmann.

Published by IMB Publishing 2015